ARABIAN MEDICINE

AND ITS INFLUENCE ON THE
MIDDLE AGES

VOLUME II

AMS PRESS
NEW YORK

ARABIAN MEDICINE

AND ITS INFLUENCE ON THE MIDDLE AGES

BY

Dr DONALD CAMPBELL

*Captain late Royal Army Medical Corps, and formerly Indian Army
Reserve of Officers, Infantry Branch*

VOL. II

LONDON
KEGAN PAUL, TRENCH, TRUBNER & CO., LTD.
BROADWAY HOUSE: 68-74 CARTER LANE, E.C.
1926

Library of Congress Cataloging in Publication Data

Campbell, Donald Edward Henry, 1883-
  Arabian medicine and its influence on the Middle Ages.

  Original ed. issued in series: Trubner's oriental
series.
  Bibliography: v. 2, p.
  1. Medicine, Arabic. 2. Medicine, Medieval.
I. Title. [DNLM: WZ70 JA7 C2a 1926F]
R143.C3 1973   610'.9'02   74-180330
ISBN 0-404-56235-3

Reprinted from the edition of 1926, London
First AMS edition published in 1973
Manufactured in the United States of America

International Standard Book Number:
Complete Set: 0-404-56235-3
Volume II: 0-404-56237-X

AMS PRESS INC.
NEW YORK, N. Y.   10003

CONTENTS

PAGE

APPENDIX I: LATIN TRANSLATORS OF THE ARABIC WORK   3

APPENDIX II: AN INVESTIGATION OF THE DATE AND
AUTHORSHIP OF THE LATIN VERSIONS OF
THE WORKS OF GALEN 13

BIBLIOGRAPHY 221

INDEX 229

ARABIAN MEDICINE

AND

ITS INFLUENCE IN THE MIDDLE AGES

VOLUME II

APPENDIX I

LATIN TRANSLATORS OF THE ARABIC WORKS

Here is set forth an alphabetical list of the Latin Translators of the Middle Ages who rendered into Latin, of varying degrees of accuracy, the medical and philosophical works of the Arabians. After each name will be found a brief note of the works translated. The information contained in this section, together with the vastly superior number of Arabic MSS. described in Chapter II of this work (*q.v.*), undeniably illustrates the fact that what was known as *Arabian Medicine*, or to be more precise, " Sarracenic studies " during the Middle Ages, was but a poor shadow of the Hellenism of the Mahomedans.

The other significant points that have a bearing on the purpose underlying the publication of this book, are that the Latin MSS. of the Greek medical works are later than the Arabic, and that the Latin renderings from the Arabic are executed with less skill and knowledge than from the Greek (or Syriac) into Arabic. In addition, the bulk of the mediaeval Latin translations are *older* than the extant Greek texts (which are mostly of the fifteenth century).

Abraham of Tortosa translated the *De Simplicibus* of Serapion Junior, and the *Liber Servitoris* of Albucasis.

Accursius of Pistoja translated the Arabic MSS. of Galen (from the Arabic of Ḥunayn).

Alfonso of Toledo translated the tract *De separatione primi principii* which was ascribed to Averroës.

Alfred the Englishman (" Alphiatus " in the MSS.) (*c.* 1200–27) translated the *De plantis* of Nicholas of Damascus, and the pseudo-Aristotelian work *De vegetabilibus*, which was probably from the pen of Isḥāq ibn Ḥunayn.

Andreas assisted Michael Scot in his translations from the Arabic.

Andreas Alpagus (or Alphagus) Bellnensis (d. 1520), translated the *Canon* and the *De medicinis cordialibus et Cantica* of Avicenna ; the *De Thericca* of Averroës (published in the Opp. Aristotelis in 1552 and 1560). He also translated the following works of Avicenna : *De anima, De Mahad,* i.e. *De dispositione seu loco, ad quem revertitur homo, Aphorismi de amina, De diffinitionibus et quæsitis, De divisione scientiarum* (published in Venice in 1546). The *Practica* of Serapion, *Al-Qifti* of Ta'rikh al-'Hukama : *De correctione errorum qui accidunt in regimine sanitatis, De lapidibus prætiosis et pleraque alia, De removendis nocumentis . . . ex errore.* The *De malis limonis* of Albe'thar, and *De syrupo acetoso* of (?) Avicenna.

Antonius Frachantius Vicentinus translated Avicenna's *Sufficientia.*

Armengaud (d. 1314) translated into Latin from the Hebrew versions of the Arabic works. Among those known as Avicenna's *Canticum* with Averroës' commentary (*c.* 1280 or 1284) ; and Ḥunayn's Arabic versions of Galen. He also translated into Latin the MSS. of Maimonides (" De regimine sanitatis ad soldanum," MS. Caio-Gonv. Camb. n. 178).

Arnold of Villanova translated (d. 1312) Avicenna's *De viribus cordis* (? 1282), revised in the Latin by Andreas Alpagus (d. 1520). The *De physicis ligaturis* of Kosta ibn Luka which was probably copied from Galen (see Steinschneider's *Die europäischen aus dem Arabischen,* Wien, 1904, p. 6).

Berengarius of Valentia translated Albucasis' *Dictio de Cibariis.*

Bonacossa (a Jew) of Padua, translated Averroës' *Colliget.*

Constantine the African translated :—

De oculis (doubtfully ascribed to Ḥunayn).

Megatechne (or *De methodo medendi, sive de ingenio sanitatis abbreviata*).

De mulierum morbis sive de matrice (gynecia).

De humana natura (or *membris principal, De compagine membrorum*).

De interioribus membris (this is identical with the Arabic version by Hubaysh ibn el-Hasan of Galen's *De locis affectis*, which again is nothing more or less than first and longer part of the Syriac Book of Medicine (see vol. i, page 13, footnote 1)).

Commentary on Hippocrates' Aphorisms (from the Arabic of Ḥunayn or Hubaysh and another).

Microtechne (or Ars Parva); this work bearing the title *De spermate* is in manuscript at Oxford (Merton, 213–19, and Balliol 231–4).

Disput. Platonis cum Hippocrate (from the Arabic of Hubaysh).

All the preceding are described by Steinschneider as Constantine's translations of the pseudo-Galenic works.

Hartmann's Thesis, *Die Literatur von Früh-und Hoch-salerno*, which is a valuable and original contribution to the study of history, contains a complete list of the Latin works of Constantine that are extant (see vol. i, p. 123).

Daniel de Morley (an Englishman) (*c*. 1190), a student at Oxford, Paris and Toledo, translated a number of works from Arabic into Latin.

David the Jew, who lived between 1228 and 1245, translated Rhazes (Albubator) into Latin.

Demetrius translated the pseudo-Galenic work *De oculis*.

Dominicus (see under the name Gundisalvi).

Drogon or Azogont translated the *De pluviis imbribus et ventis et de æris mutatione* of al-Kindi (Venice, 1507, Paris, 1540).

Farragut (or Faradj ben Salem) translated the pseudo-Galenic work *De medicinis expertis* from the Arabic of Honein, the *Tacuini ægritudinum* of Byngezla, the *Chirurgia* of pseudo-Mesuë, and the *Continens* of Rhazes.

Franciscus de Macerata translated the *Metaphysica* of Avicenna.

G. under this letter we have the Latin translation *De simplici medicina* (? 1258) from the Arabic *al-Gafiki*. G. was a son of magister Johannes of Lerida and MSS. of his translation are at Berne and Munich.

Gerard of Cremona's translations from Arabic into Latin include the following :—

Alexander's *De (motu et) tempore* (original MSS. are lost).

     ,,   *De sensu.*

     ,,   *De eo quod augmentum et incrementum fiant in forma et non in yle* (from the Arabic of Sa'id of Damascus, MS. Escur. 294–10).

     ,,   *De intellectu et intellecto* (from the Arabic of Isḥāq ibn Ḥunayn) ; published in 1501, and at other times without the name of the translator.

     ,,   *De unitate* (MS. Par. 6443).

     ,,   *Apollonius.*

     ,,   *Archimedes* (probably from the Arabic of Thabit). MSS. are at Turin and Paris.

Aristotle's *Analyt. poster* (from the Arabic of Matta).

     ,,   *De expositione bonitatis puræ* (from an anonymous Arabic translation).

     ,,   *De naturali auditu* (from the Arab. Quellen).

     ,,   *De Cœlo et mundo* (the Arab translator is uncertain).

     ,,   *De causis proprietatum* or *De proprietatibus elementorum tract I*. Tract II, credited to Gerard, has not been found.

     ,,   *De generatione et corruptione* (Arab. translator uncertain).

     ,,   *Lib. Meteorum. III Tract* (from the Arabic of Ja'hja ibn al-Batrik).

Aristotle's *Lib. Lapidum.*

,,   *Autolykos (De sphœra motu).* (Arabic translator uncertain, probably rendered into Arabic by Ḥunayn and corrected by Thabit.) MSS. in Paris and Venice.

Diocles' *De speculis comburentibus* (this is a fragment out of *Eutokios).* (From the Arabic of Thabit ibn Kurra.)

Euclid's *Elemente,* XV books.   This work was translated into Arabic by Isḥāq ibn Ḥunayn, Thabit ibn Kurra, 'Hadjdjadj ibn Jusuf, and Kosta ibn Luka.

Galen's *De elementis* (from the Arabic of Ḥunayn).

,,   Commentary on Hippocrates' Regimen acutorum III Tr. (from the Arabic of Ḥunayn).

,,   *De secretis ad Monteum* (from the Arabic of Ḥunayn).

,,   *De complexionibus (temperamente)* (from the Arabic of Ḥunayn).

,,   *De Malitia complexionis diversæ* (from the Arabic of Ḥunayn).

,,   *De simplici medicina Tr. I–IV* (from the Arabic of Ḥunayn or Ja'hja ibn al-Batrik ?).

,,   *De crisi* (the MSS. are extant).

,,   Commentary on Hippocrates' Prognostica (from the Arabic of Ḥunayn and not from the Latin rendering of Constantine).

,,   *Tegni* (Ars parva) (from the Arabic of Ḥunayn). This work was published at Venice in 1496, 1521, 1523, 1527, and numerous MSS. were issued under the name of Haly Eben Rodan, or Rodoham, without the mention of Gerard's name.

Hippocrates' *Lib. veritatis* or *Sapientiæ* (there is an Arabic MS. by Ja'hjà ibn al-Batrik and also a version by Ḥunayn).

,,   *Regimen acutorum.*

,,   *Prognost.* with Galen's commentary.

,,   *De ascensionibus* (from the Arabic of Kosta Ibn Luka, or Isḥāq ibn Ḥunayn).

Menelaos' *De figuris spericis* (from the Arabic of Ḥunayn).

Ptolemy's *Almagest* (both the Latin MSS. extant, Cantabr. St. Petri 51 ; s. xiii–xiv, f. 115*b*, and Monac. 276 ; s. xiv, f. 83 contain the commentary of Haly).

Themistius' Commentary on Arsitotle's *Analyt. Poster.* (MS. Par. 16097).

Theodosius' *De sp(h)æris* (from the Arabic of Kosta and Thabit).

,,   *De locis habitibilus* (from the Arabic of Kosta).

The following are Gerard's Latin translations from the works of the medical writers of Islam :—

Aben-Guefit : *Kitab al Wisad* known in Latin translation as *Liber Abenguefiti Medicinarum simplicium et ciborum.* The publications are Argentor 1537 and Venice 1558.

Avicenna : The *Canon.*

Al-Farabi : *De syllogismo.* This work is an elaboration of Aristotle's Logic, but both the original Arabic and the Latin versions have yet to be safely ascertained.

,,   *Distinctio super librum Aristotelis de naturali auditu.*

,,   *De scientiis* (MS. Escurial 643). Gerard's translation may be seen in Paris (Suppl. lat. 49).

Alfragani : *De aggregationibus scientiæ stellarum*, etc.

Isaac Judæus : *De elementis.*

,,   *De descriptione rerum et diffinitionibus.*

,,   *De aspectibus.* MS. Oxf. Corp. Christi, 254–9.

,,   *De quinque essentiis.*

,,   *De sompno (somno) et visione.*

,,   *De (rerum) gradibus medicinarum.*

Rhazes : *Liber ad Almansorem.*

,,   *Liber divisionum.*

,,   *Liber introductorius in medicina parvus.*

,,   *De ægritudinibus junctuarum.*

Serapion Junior : *Breviarium.*

Thabit ben Korra : *De figura alchata (sectore).*

Zahravius (Albucasis) : The *Chirurgia.* The MS. Par.
10236 is illustrated with figures. Gerard
also translated the *Liber Servitoris.*

The anonymous Arabic works translated by Gerard of Cremona
include the following :—

Practica geometriæ which is identical with the
geometry of Abu Bekr.

Lib. Divinitatis (primus) de LXX on alchemy.

De aluminibus et salibus (said to have been
written by Rhazes), as is also *Lib. lumen
luminum* (MSS. Paris 6514–12, 7156–7
and 7158–15) which were translated by
Gerard of Cremona.

Gundisalvi translated the *Sufficientia* of Avicenna (*Avicennæ
Opera*, 1495, 1500, and 1508).

Herman the German, who is said to have been a teacher of Roger
Bacon, lived between the years 1240 and 1260. His writings
are uncertain but he is ascribed with the Latin translation
of Averroës' commentary on the rhetoric and poetry of
Aristotle (1256), the commentary of the ethics of Aristotle

(1240), a book entitled *Summa quorundam Alexandrinorum* (1243 or 1244), and al-Farabi's *Declaratio compendiosa . . . super libris Rhetoricorum Arist.*

Jacobus Sylvius translated two books of the *De simplicibus*, book three (*De antidotis*) being doubtfully ascribed to Mesuë Junior.

Jambolinus Cremonensis (probably the same as Johannes Bonus) translated extracts from the work of Gege the son of Algazel, from Arabic into Latin.

John of Capua (d. 1162 or 1177) translated the *Regimen* (?) and the *De causis accidentium apparentium domino et magnifico soldaro, etc.* of Maimonides from the Hebrew into Latin. Though not of direct interest to us, but of value in the study of the history of folk-lore in Europe, it may be mentioned here that John of Capua translated the *Kilila and Dimna* of Bidpai. He is the John of Campania who translated the *Theisir* of Avenzoar (MS. Par. 6948).

Johannes Hispalensis (Avendeath or John of Toledo). His translations were chiefly of Arabic works on astronomy and astrology rather than on philosophy. He translated the pseudo-Aristotelian work *Epistola de conservatione corporis humani, i.e. secretum secretorum,* from the Arabic of Ja'hja ibn al-Batrik. He also translated into Latin Avicenna's *Sufficientia* (Arab. *Schafa*), *De anima VI naturalium, Metaphysica,* or *Philosophia prima, sive scientia divina* (MS. Par. 6443), *De cœlo et mundo.* His other Latin translations include Kosta ibn Luka's *Differentia inter animam et spiritum,* al-Farabi's *De scientiis, sive lib. Gundisalvi de divisione philosophiæ,* Avicebron's (Gabirol) *Fons vitæ,* al-Gazzali's three books on logic, metaphysics, and physic, al-Kindi's *De intellectu (et intellecto),* Thabit ibn Kurra's *De imaginibus astronomicis.*

Johannes Lodoycus Tetrapharmacos translated (1198) the *Antidotarium* of Albucasis (MSS. are at Venice and Vienna).

Kalonymos translated (1328) Averroës' *Destructio destructionis* (MSS. are Vat. 2434, and St. Marco, Ven. Valentinelli V, 416, n. 64).

Manfred de Monte translated *De simplicibus* from the Arabic ?

Marcus of Toledo, who is known only from his own works, translated into Latin the following of Galen from the Arabic texts :—

> *De tactu pulsus.*
> *De motu musculorum (membrorum).*
> *De utilitate.*
> *De motibus liquidis (lucidis, fluidis, difficilibus).*

The four preceding works were from the Arabic of Ḥunayn. Marcus also translated into Latin the *Isagoge ad Tegni Galeni* of Joanittius (or Ḥunayn), and Hippocrates' *De aëre, aquis, etc.* (MS. Vienna 11, 57, n. 2328 *b*).

Michael Scot was assisted in his Latin translations of the Arabic works by the Jew Andreas ; their works include the following Latin translations from the Arabic :—

Aristotle's *De cœlo et mundo,* with Averroës' commentary.
> ,,   *De generatione et corruptione.*
> ,,   *De animalibus.*
> ,,   *De anima.*
> ,,   *De sensu et sensato* (from Averroës' paraphrasis).
> ,,   *Metaphysica.*

Averroës' *De substantia orbis.*

Moses of Palermo (1277) translated the pseudo-Hippocratic work *De curationibus infirmitatum œquorum,* of which two Italian versions containing extracts were issued in the thirteenth century.

Paravicious (or Paravicinus or Patavinus), a physician of Venice (1280), translated the *Theisir* of Avenzoar.

Peter of Abano, who lived between the years 1253 and 1316, translated the Arabic version of the Hippocratic writing *Astrologia*.

Robert the Englishman prepared a Latin translation of al-Kindi's *De judiciis* and *De proportione et proportionalitate*.

Simon Januensis (*c.* 1290), together with the Jew Abraham Tortuosiensis, translated the *Synonyma*, the *De simplicibus* of Serapion Junior, which was a collection from Dioscorides and Galen (Venice 1497, 1550), Lugd. 1525, Argentor, 1531. He also translated the *Liber servitoris* book xxviii (book xxvii in the edition published in 1589, but the material on the preparation of medicines is identical).

Simon (son of Seth) of Antioch (*c.* 1080), translated *Kalila and Dimna* from the Arabic.

Stephen of Antioch (1127) translated *Al-Kitabu'l-Maliki* of Haly Abbas, and Latin editions were published at Venice (1492) and Lyons (1523).

Stephen of Lerida (1233) translated *Liber fiduciæ de simplicibus medicinis* (MS. at Munich, see Rohlf's Deutsch. Archiv. für Gesch. der Med. 11, 1879).

Theodorus, according to *MS. Amplon 352 Fol.*, presents us with a repetition of the prologue of Averroës' Commentary on Physic, which begins " Intentio mea in hoc libro ".

Witelo the Pole translated the *Optics* of Alhazen.

APPENDIX II

AN INVESTIGATION OF THE DATE AND AUTHORSHIP OF THE LATIN VERSIONS OF THE WORKS OF GALEN

In the ensuing pages I propose reconstructing the Galenic Library as it was known in the Middle Ages.

All the known works of Galen that were translated into Latin will be placed under their respective titles, and the dates will be shown as far as the material at our disposal permits. While it is intended to keep in mind the Latin versions as the principal purpose of my research, the Greek, Syriac, Arabic, and Hebrew texts will be referred to in so far as they have a direct bearing on this attempt to place before the reader the Galenic works as understood by the Mediaeval Scholastics.

The principal interest of this catalogue of the Galenic Library lies in the fact that it gives us a reflected picture of the great thought movements of the intellectual Middle Ages, at a time when the transition from the mediaeval to the modern world took place, with all it meant to mankind from the viewpoint of its spiritual activity with special reference to the revival of classical arts and letters.

It is much to be regretted that while Aristotle and other ' giants ' of classical times have been, and are, studied with great assuetude, Galen and the medical philosophers have been abandoned to a mere handful of research workers who are scattered from Leipzig and Vienna on the one side, to Washington on the other.

An investigation of the individual manuscripts may yet reveal an aspect of the classics and mediaeval thought that up to the present is hidden from us, and for this reason alone the writer felt sufficiently enthusiastic to compile the data here given.

The arrangement of the appendix will be as follows. The title of the work, together with its name in Greek, where such exist, will be followed by a note on all the manuscripts that are known ; then will follow a list of the Latin MSS. and translations, with notes on each.

ABBREVIATIONS

An asterisk after the MS. indicates that it is an abbreviation of an original.

The letter D. = Op. Gal. (Giunta ed., 1528), thus : D. I, f. 60 = Giunta edition (1528), tome 1, folio 60.

The letter C. = Operum Galeni (copy of which is in the British Museum, and in the writer's private library), thus : C. III, f. 818 = ed. Lugduni, 1550, tome 3, folio 818. This edition is unknown to Brunet and Deschamps, Græsse, III, 8 ; Jourdan, IV, 324, mentions only ed. Lyons, 1552, in folio.

The letters [B.M.] after a Latin work indicate that the said work is in the British Museum, and the figures preceding them are the numbers in the Index Catalogue.

(1)

Opera varia

Greek, Syriac, Arabic, Hebrew, and Latin MSS. are known.
Latin MSS.

Cambridge :   Cantabr. St. Petri 1862

Einsiedeln :   Bibl. monast. 304 ; s. ix

Leyden :   Vossian. 2157

Osimo :   nr. 51 ; s. xvi

Padua :   Bibl. Ordinis Eremitanorum (Lat. ?).   Whereabouts not known

Paris :   Bibl. Univ. 125 ; s. xiii (Libri xviii de medicina)

(2)

Γαληνοῦ παραφράστου τοῦ Μηνοδότου προτρεπτικὸς λόγος
ἐπὶ τὰς τέχνας

Galeni paraphrastæ Menodoti suasoria ad artes oratio

A Greek and Latin MS. have been described. The following is
the Latin MS. Berens. lat. N. 128 ; a. 1565 (impr.)

Latin translations

— C. V, f. 1, second part. (Inscr. Claudii Galeni Paraphrastæ Menodoti filii suasoria ad artes oratio, Ludouico
Bellisario Medico Mutinensi Interprete)

— The three following publications contain both the Greek
and Latin texts. Galeni . . . suasoria ad artes oratio. See
CALLIMACHUS. Callimachi hymni et epigrammata &c. 1741.
8° *997 h. 6* [B.M.]

— Γαληνοῦ προτρεπτικὸς ἐπὶ τὰς τέχνας, Galeni adhortatio
ad artes. Cum sua annotatione et versione D. Erasmi edidit
A. Willet. Lugduni Batavorum. 1812. 8° *8408 c. c. 2* [B.M.]

— Κλανδίον Γαληνοῦ . . . Τῶν σωζομένων Τινά, Claudii
Galeni . . . opuscula varia [*i.e.* Oratio Suasoria ad Artes.
Quod optimus Medicus idem et philosophus. De optimo
docendi genere. De sectis. De optima secta. De dignoscendis
animi affectibus. De dignoscendis animi erratis. De substantia naturalium facultatum. — Quod animi mores sequantur
temperamentum corporis]. A. . . . T. Goulstono . . . Græca
recensita, mendisque . . . repurgata, et in linguam Latinam
. . . traducta . . . Accessere ab eodem variæ lectiones, et
annotationes criticæ. Londini. 1640. 4° *540 f. 7* [B.M.]

(3)

περὶ ἀρίστης διδασκαλίας
Quod optima doctrina

There is a Greek MS. at Florence.

Latin translations

Giunta ed. (1528), 1, fol. 18

(4)

ὅτι ὁ ἄριστος ἰατρὸς καὶ φιλοσοφος

Quod optimus medicus sit etiam philosophus

Of the MSS. only the Greek survive (at Florence, Paris, Rome, and Venice). There are Greek MSS. said to be in England, though their whereabouts are not known.

Latin translations.

— C. V, f. 17–20, second part (Inscr. Claud. Galeni quid optimus Medicus est, eundum esse Philosophum ; Ludouico Bellisario Medico Mutinensi Interprete)

— Claudii Galeni . . . opuscula varia (London, 1640), contains a Latin translation together with the Greek text freshly translated into Latin and published by Goulstone (*540 f. 7* B.M.). The Latin version in this edition is inscribed '' Quod optimus Medicus idem et philosophus ''.

(5)

περὶ αἱρέσεων τοῖς εἰσαγομένοις

De sectis ad eos qui introducuntur

Greek, Arabic, and Latin MSS. are known.

Latin MSS.

  Bourges : Biturigens. 299 (247) ; s. xiv, f. 105
  Cesena : Malatest. D. XXV, 1 ; s. xiii, f. 7
                 D. XXV, 2 ; s. xiii
                 S. V, 4 ; s. xiv
  Erfurt : Amplon. F. 280 ; s. xiv in f. 46
  Leipzig : Lipsiens. Repos. med. 1, 22 ; s. —
  Montpellier : Montepass. (École de méd.) 18 ; s. xiii
  Munich : Monacens. 5 ; s. xiv, f. 12
                     490 ; a. 1488–1503
  Paris : Parisin. 6865 ; s. xv, f. 81, 84

Rome : Palat. 1090 ; s. —, f. 1
          1094 ; s. xiv, f. 544
     Urbin. 247 ; s. xiv, f. 52 ᵛ
     Vatic. 2376 ; s. —, f. 199
          2389 ; s. —, f. 1

Latin Translations

— Claudii Galeni . . . opuscula varia (London, 1640), contains both the Greek and Latin texts.

— C. V, f. 51 (Ludouico Bellisario Mutinensi Interprete) Inc. Id sane quo medicina intendit, sanitas est. Expl. præsentibus finem imposnam.

(6)

πρὸς Θρασύβουλον περὶ τῆς ἀρίστης αἱρέσεως

De optima secta ad Thrasybulum liber

Greek and Latin MSS. are known.

Latin MSS.

Cesena : Malatest. D. XXV, 2 ; s. xiii (Henr. regi a
                 Burgundione transl.)
Munich : Monacens. e bibl. Hartm. Schedelii Incunab. c.a.
            2410 (Capp. 1–8 a Nicol. Rhegin. transl.)

Latin translations

— D. I, f. 18

— C. V, f. 63 (amended) 96 (Junio Paulo Crasso Patauino Interprete)
         Inc. Singula medica præcepta
         Expl. quibus libere atque explicate proprios usus
            exhibeant

— Claudii Galeni . . . opuscula varia (*Brit. Mus. 540 f. 7*) (London, 1640) contains both the Greek and Latin texts of " De optima secta ".

(7)

πρὸς Πατρόφιλον περὶ συστάσεως ἰατρικῆς

De constitutione artis medicæ ad Patrophilum liber

Greek and Latin MSS. survive.

Latin MSS.

Angers : Andecavens. 461 (446) ; s. xvi, f. 98
Dresden : Dresd. Db. 92, 93 ; s. xv, f. 295d
Paris : Parisin. 7023 ; s. xvi, No. 3

Latin translations

— D. I, f. 20 (Nicholao de Regio interpr.)

— C. V, f. 113–34 (Bartholomæo Syluanio Salonensi Interprete)
 Inscr. Claudii Galeni de medicæ artis constitutione
 Inc. Quoniam diuino quodam preditus instinctu
  mihi videris, Patrophile . . .
 Expl. eorum scopos confecit curationis

— Claudi Galeni Pergameni de constitutione artis medicæ
liber, Jano Antoniaco interprete. Parisiis, 1531. 8° *540 d. 7
(2)* [B.M.]

— Galeni de constitutione artis medicæ, ad Patrophilum
V. Trincavellio interprete. Parisiis, 1547. 8° *774 b. 30 (3)*
[B.M.]

— In Galeni librum de constitutione artis medicæ tabulæ
et commentarii : per T. Zuinggerum . . . (C. Galeni de constitutione artis medicæ . . . V. Trincavelio interprete) . . .
Accessit . . . index. Basileæ, 1561 fol. *539 k. 7 (3)* [B.M.]

The text precedes the Tabulæ.

— F. Valleriolæ . . . commentarii in librum Galeni de
constitutione artis medicæ. (With the text.) Lugduni, 1577.
8° *540 d. 18* [B.M.]

(8)

Ars medica

Greek, Syriac, Arabic, Hebrew, and Latin MSS. are known.

Latin MSS.

Autun : Augustodunens. 70 ; s. xiv, No. 3 (c. Comm. Haly)

Auxerre : Antissiodurens. 240 (203) ; s. xii, f. 49 (Expl. in medio cap. quod inscr. De parvo hepate et augusto)

Bamberg : Bibl. publ. 536 (L. III, 12) ; s. xii (Desunt quattuor ult. §§)

      537 (L. III, 11) ; s. xii

      1331 (L. III, 20) ; s. xiii in (In art. parvam notæ)

Basle : Basil. D. I, 6 ; s. —

Breslau : Vratisl. bibl. acad. Ac. IV, F. 27* ; s. xv, f. 1–261 (Tres. quæstt. sec. Jacobum de Latere de Forlivio)

     Kornian. 21 ; s. xiv

Bruges : Bibl. publ. 474 ; s. xiii–xv

Budapest : nr. 41 ; s. xiv, f. 1 (Tres quæstt. sec. Jacobum de la Torre de Forlivio. Inc. et expl. mutil.)

Cambridge : Cantabr. Coll. caii 59 ; s. xiv, f. 251 (c. Comm. Haly) 962 ; s. —

     Corp. Christi 364 ; s. xiii, f. 55

     St. Johann D. 24 ; s. xiii (Expl. orationem in eis)

     E. 29 ; s. xiii

     Pembroke 2055 ; s. — (Comm.)

     St. Petri 14 ; s. xiv, f. 101 (c. C. Haly)

        248; s. xiii, f. 1, 226 et s. xii/xiii, f. iv, 34 (Expl. nec indigestionem vero)

        1866 ; s. —

     St. Trinitat O. I. 59 ; s. xii/xiii, f. 35 (42)

     Univ. J. i, II, 5 ; s. xiv, f. 17–24 (c. C. Haly. Expl. in complexione eius)

Chartres : Autricens. 278 (258 et 666) ; s. xiv, f. 54 (c. Comm.
               Haly)
            286 (342) ; s. xiv, f. 148 (c. C. Haly)
            287 (343)* ; s. xiv (Anon. Comm. in
             art. parva.)

Clermont-Ferrand : nr. 213 (180) ; s. xiii, f. 50
                214 (181) ; s. xiii, f. 19 (corresponds to
                 Cantabr. St. Joh. D. 24)

Copenhagen : Harmiens. bibl. reg. 3479 ; s. xv, ex. f. 109

Cues : Bibl. Nic. Cusani med. 3 ; s. xii, xiii, No. 3 (Gal.
                 " regimentum " c. C. Haly)
              4 ; s. xii, xiii, No. 3

Dresden : Dresd. Db. 92, 93 ; s. xv, f. 108c

Dublin : Coll. Trinit. 403 ; s. xvi

Durham : Eccl. Dunelm. C. IV, 4 ; s. xiii in. ? f. 17

Edinburgh : Advocates' Library W. 5, 23 (18, 6, 11) ; s. xii,
      ex. — xiii (corresponds to Cantabr. S. Joh. D. 24)

Einsiedeln : Bibl. monast. 32 ; s. xii, f. 311

Erfurt : Amplon. F. 258 ; s. xiii–xiv, f. 35
          F. 289* ; s. xiv in. f. 60
          Q. 173 ; s. xiii, f. 47 (corresponds to
             Cantabr. St. Joh. D. 24)
          Q. 178 ; s. xiii, f. 6 (c. notulis Comm. Haly,
             Thaddei, Bartholomei et Johannis de
             S. Amando)
          Q. 182 ; s. xiii, f. 33

Eton : Bibl. Coll. 127 ; s. xiv, f. 183 (c. C. Haly)

Florence : Laurent. plut. 29, 27* ; s. xv, p. 44 (Anon. in art.
                   parvam quæstt.)
           73, 10 ; s. xv, f. 1
           73, 21 ; s. xiv, f. 34
           73, 28 ; s. xiii, f. 46

Glasgow : Hunterian. T. 1, 1 ; s. xiv (c. C. Haly)

Gotha : Herg. Bibl. 63 (Membr. II, 144) ; s. —, f. 144

Hamburg : Uffenbach. 107 ; a 1431, No. 6

Laon : Laudemens. 413 ; s. xiv, No. 3 (c. C. Haly)
              416 ; s. xiii, No. 7 (c. C. Haly)

Leipzig : Lipsiens. bibl. univ. Repos. med. I. 28 ; s. —
        (c. C. Haly)
           II, 26 ; s. —

Leyden : Vossian, 2002 ; s. —

London : Addit. (Brit. Mus.) 22, 668 ; s. xiii, xiv, f. 18 (corre-
        sponds to Cantabr. St. Joh. D. 24)

        Arundel. 162 ; s. xiv, f. 51 (c. C. Haly)
               215 ; s. xiv in. f. 136 (corresponds to
                  Cantabr. St. Joh. D. 24)

        Harleian. 3140 ; s. xiii, f. 7 (corresponds to
            Cantabr. St. Joh. D. 24)

        Sloan. 1124 ; s. xiii, f. 11 (corresponds to
            Cantabr. St. Joh. D. 24)
             1610 ; s. xiv, f. 7 (corresponds to Cantabr.
            St. Joh. D. 24)

        Medical Society. Wa 2 ; s. xiii, f. 4 (Inc. mutil. ;
            Labent terminos. Quæcumque vero.
            Expl. propriis conscriptionibus)

Madrid : Matrit. bibl. nac. 1407 (ol. L, 59) ; s. xiv, f. 105
        (c. C. H.)
        1408 (ol. L, 61) ; s. xv, f. 120 (c. C. H.)

Metz : Mediomatric. 177 ; s. xiv, No. 5 (c. Comm.)

Montpellier : Montepass. (École de méd.) 182 ; s. xiv, No. 5
                            (c. C. Haly)
                      188 ; s. xiv, No. 6
                            (c. C. Haly)

Montecassino : Casinens. 397* ; s. xiii, p. 1 (Expositiio in
        art. parva)

Munich : Monac.   31 ; a. 1302, f. 134 (c. C. Haly)

168 ; s. xiv, f. 133 (c. C. Haly)

270 ; s. xiv, f. 101 (c. C. Haly)

465 ; a. 1503, f. 2 (Apogr. libri Venetiis
a. 1503 editi)

692* ; a. 1463, f. 197

3512 (Aug. civ, 12) ; a. 1300, f. 298 (c. C.
Haly)

4395 (Aug. S. Ubr. 95) ; s. xv, f. 129

4622 (Bened. 122) ; s. xi–xiii, f. 79 (mutil.)

11322 (Polling. 22) ; s. xiv, f. 6

13034 (Rat. civ, 34) ; s. xiv, f. 12 (c. C.
Haly)

13111 (Rat. civ, 111) ; s. xiii, f. 30

13147 (Rat. civ, 147) ; s. xv, f. 1 (Comm.
in a.p.)

19425 (Teg. 1425) ; s. xiii, f. 57 (Comm. Haly)

Orleans : Aurelianens. 284 (238) ; s. xiv, f. 75

Oxford : Coll. Omn. Animar.   71 ; s. xiv in. f. 113 (c. C. Haly)
1430 ; s. —

Bodleian 1052 ; s. —

2753 ; s. — (Comm.)

Canonician (Bodl.) 272 ; s. xiv, ex. f. 81 (Expl. in
1, III, c. 214)

Laudian. 65 ; s. xiii, f. 65

106 ; s. xiii, f. 18

Coll. St. Joh. Bapt. 10 ; s. xiii ex. f. 99 (c. C. Haly)

Merton 220 ; s. xiv, f. 110 (c. C. H. Expl. magis
completum est)

221 ; s. xiv, f. 161 (c. C. anon. et c. C. H.)

222 ; s. xiv, f. 5 (Expl. corresponds to Lond.
Med. Soc. Wa 2a et f. 21)

255 ; s. xiv in. f. 11b

Norvic. 1130 ; s. —
Coll. Novi 166 ; s. xiii ex. f. 40
    170 ; s. xiv, f. 17 (c. C. Haly)
Univ. 89 (c. C. Haly)

Padua : Bibl. S. Augustin, ed. lævam plut. XXVI (whereabouts not known)

Paris : Bibl. de l'Arsenal 1080 ; s. xiv, f. 29 (abbreviat.)
Bibl. Facult. Med ? ; s. xv
Bibl. Mazarin 1289 ; s. xiii (Frgm. Comm.)
Parisin. 6846 ; s. xiv, No. 4 (c. C. anon.)
    6856 ; s. xv, No. 2 (Comm.)
    6868 ; s. xiv, No. 4
    6869 ; s. xiv, No. 7 (c. C. Haly)
    6870 ; s. xiv, No. 6
    6871 ; s. xiv, No. 7
    6871A ; s. xiv, No. 5
    7029 ; s. xiv, No. 1
    7030 ; s. xiv, No. 1 (Frgm. in introd. Johannitii)
    7030A ; s. xiv, No. 4 (c. C. Haly)
    14390 ; s. xiv, f. 5
    15457 ; s. xiii, f. 1 (c. C. Haly)
    16174 ; s. xiii, f. 117
    16176 ; s. xiii, f. 26
    16177 ; s. xiii, f. 91 (c. C. Haly)
    16178 ; s. xiv, f. 63 (c. Comm.)
    16188 ; s. xiii, f. 213 (c. C. Haly)
    17157 ; s. xiv, f. 137 (c. C. Haly)
    18500 ; s. xiii, ex. f. 16 (c. C. Haly)
    nouv. acq. 1480 ; s. xiv, f. 58 (c. C. Haly)
       1481 ; s. xiv, f. 101 (c. C. Haly)
Bibl. Univ. 580 ; s. xiv (c. C. Haly)

Pavia : Bibl. Univ. 383 ; s. xv, f. 71 (c. C. Haly)

Rebdorf : Bibl. d. Augustiner-Chothorm 11 ; s. xiii
Regensburg : Bibl. urb. 68 ; s. — (c. C. Haly)
Reims : nr. 1001 ; s. xiii, f. 31
           1002 ; s. xiii, f. 10
           1003 ; s. xiv, f. 116 (c. C. Haly)
Rome : Angelic. 1456 (V. I, 11)* ; s. xv, f. 114
     Palat. 1089 ; s. —, f. 1 et 64
          1102 ; s. —, f. 117 (c. C. Haly)
          1103 ; s. —, f. 89 (c. C. Haly)
     Regin. 1270 ; s. xiv, f. 56 (c. C. Haly)
          1302 ; s. xiv, f. 54 (c. C. Haly)
          1304 ; s. —, f. 19
     Vatic. 2392* ; s. —, f. 34 (" Caput ult. quo de suis
                              operibus agit ")
          2417 ; s. —, (lib. 1)
          2461 ; s. —, f. 42 (corresponds to Cantabr.
                           St. Joh. D. 24)
          4455 ; s. —, f. 23
          6241 ; s. —, f. 34
Rouen : Rotomagens. 978 (J. 57) ; s. xiv, f. 21
S. Daniele del Friuli : nr. 145 ; s. xiv (Inscr. De conservanda
                         valetudine)
St. Gallen : Vadian. 431 ; a. 1465 (c. C. Haly)
                 432 ; s. xv, f. 228 (c. C. anon.)
St. Mihiel : nr. 37 ; s. xiv, No. — (c. C. Haly)
St. Cuer : nr. 617 ; s. xiii, No. 5
St. Quentin : nr. 104 (91) ; s. xiii, No. 5 (c. C. Haly)
Toulouse : Tolosan. 762 (I. 129) ; s. — (Comm. anon.)
Turin : Taurinens. bibl. reg. 939 (i, I. 35) ; s. xiv, f. 32
Upsala : Upsal. C. 661 ; s. xiii, f. 85 (c. C. Haly)
Utrecht : Traiectan. 679 ; s. xiv in f. 74 (c. C. Haly)
               680 ; s. xv, f. 1–38 (c. Comm. anon.)
               695 ; s. xv, f. 55–78 (Comm. anon. in art.
                            p. et f. 93–105)

Venice : Marcian. cl. XIV, 7 ; s. xiv, f. 1 (Petri Hisp. gloss.)

8 ; s. xiii, f. 1 (Lectura Ursi Laudensis super Microt. Gal.)

Vendôme : Vindocinens. 110 ; s. xv, f. 1

236* ; xv (Jacobi de Forlivio quæstt.)

Wolfenbüttel : Guelferbyt. 2194 (17, 2, Aug.) ; a. 1444, f. 137–156 (De corporis, de signis, de causis libri III)

3487 (47, 12, Aug.) ; s. xiv, f. 49–79 (Tegni Gal. de sanis et neutris corporibus et signis eorum et causis.)

Latin translations

— D. I, f. 3

— D. II, f. 281 u. 315

— C. V, f. 199 (Inscr. Claudii Galeni Ars Medicinalis, Nicolao Leoniceno Interprete)

Cap. 1. Inc. Tres sunt omnes doctrinæ, quæ ordini inhærent

Cap. 2. Inscr. Quid sit Medicina

Cap. 3. ,, Quot modis dicatur effectiuum, indicati-nuum, and susceptium

Cap. 4. ,, De corpore salubri

Cap. 5. ,, De corpore salubri

Cap. 6. ,, De corpore neutro

Cap. 7. ,, De signis salubribus

Cap. 8. ,, De signis optimæ consitutionis

Cap. 9. ,, Quot sint differentiæ partium

Cap. 10. ,, De signis cerebri

Cap. 11 to 66

Cap. 67. Inscr. De voce

Cap. 68 to 74

Cap. 75. Inscr. Quomodo cognoscantur corpora ægrotantia

Cap. 76 to 85

Cap. 86. Inscr. De venereis

Cap. 87 to 93
Cap. 94. Inscr. De obstructione
Cap. 95 to 96
Cap. 97. Inscr. De morbo secundum magnitudinem
Cap. 98. „ De morbo secundum situm
Cap. 99. „ De causis præferuatiuis
Cap. 100. „ De parte artis, quæ conualescentes reficit, and sensibus congruit

NOTE.—This Latin work was known as the *Isagoge* of Galen. Rhazes made extensive use of this Greek work, see *Opus* . . . *Galeatii de Sancta Sophia in monu tractatum libri Rhazes as regem Almansorem, etc.*, 1533 fol. [Brit. Mus. *543 g. 10 (1)*]

— Turisani monaci plus mentum in microtegni galieni cum questione ejusdem de ypostasi. (With the text.) G.L. ff. 141. madato z expesis . . . Octaviani Scoti . . . Per Bonetu Locatellu : Venetiis, pridie duo apriles (12 April), 1498 fol *I.B. 22976*, 142 leaves, the last blank. Sig. A–R in eights ; S, six leaves. Printed in double columns, 66 lines to a column [B.M.]

— Galieni . . . micro Tegni cum comento Hali Rodoham liber &c. (translated by Gerardus Cremonensis). See HUNAIN IBN ISHAK. Begin : In hoc pataro libro &c. 1487 fol. *I.B. 21384* [B.M.]

— Liber Galeni qui dicitur tegni sive ars parva. Lat. See articella. Artesala, 1491 fol. *539 h. 19* [B.M.]

— Espositio Ugonis Senensis super libros Tegni. With the text interpolated. See Hippocrates. [Aphorismi, Latin.] Expositio Ugonis . . . super aphorismos Hippocratis &c. 1498 fol. *539 i. 14 (1–3)* [B.M.]

— Summes candidissime lector animo q. libentissimo interpretatione Jacobi Forlivienois in tres libros Thegni Gal. cum questionibus ejusdem . . . correctione additionibusq . . . H. tropilli de Oleariis de Verona . . . (With the text interpolated) G.L. Few MS. notes. Venetiis, 1508 fol. *539 i. 4 (2)* [B.M.]

— Liber primus (—tertius) Tegni, Lat. See HUNAIN IBN ISHAK. Liber Hysagoge &c. 1510 ?. 8° *539 c. 34* [B.M.]

— Turisani monaci plusquam comentum in microtegni Galieni (with the text, Lat.) Cum questione ejusdem (Turisani) de Ypostasi. G.L. Venetiis, 1512 fol. *540 h. 4* [B.M.]

— (Another copy) *I.B. 23231 (2)* [B.M.]

— (Another edition) Plusquam commentum &c. Venetiis, 1519 fol. *540 h. 5* [B.M.]

— (Another edition). Plusquam commentum in parvam Galeni Artem Turisani Florentini . . . cum duplici textus interpretatione, antiqua scilicet, et Leoniceni et ejusdem (Turisani) libello De hypostasi, opus . . . quod olim quidem J.M. Rota . . . pluribus auxit et emendavit ; nunc vero . . . recognitum . . . additio quibusdam . . . denuo imprimendum curavimus. Ea autem sunt Hali, qui eandem Galeni artem primus exposuit Joannitii ad eandem introductio ; Gentilis, qui primum ejusdem artis librum partim explicando, partim dubitando declaravit ; N. Leoniceni quæstio de tribus doctrinis &c. Venetiis, 1557 fol. *540 h. 6* [B.M.]

— Expositio Ugonis Senensis super libros Tegni Galeni (with a Latin version of the text). G.L. MS. notes. Venetiis, 1518 fol. *7305 g. 17* [B.M.]

Printed in double columns.

— Libri Tres Tegni antique translationis ; translatione L. Laurentiani. See Articella. Articella nuperrime impressa &c. 1519. 8° *544 b. 8* [B.M.]

— 1525. 8° *544 b. 9* [B.M.]

— 1534. 8° *544 b. 10* [B.M.]

— Thaddei Florentini . . . in Claudii Galeni Microtechnen comentarii secude editionis, emaculati . . . studio T.D. Polii &c. Neapoli, 1522 fol. *C. 66 g. 11* [B.M.]

— In tribus libris Microtechni expositio (with the text). See BENZO (U.) Senensis. Ugonis opera &c. 1523 fol. *539 i. 15* [B.M.]

—   Ars Medicinalis interprete N. Leoniceno. See Hippocrates
—[Two or more works—Lat.] Hippocrates de Natura Humana,
A. Brentio interprete &c. 1524. 16° *539 a. 16 (5)* [B.M.]

—   Another edition. See Hippocrates [Two or more works.]
Hippocratis ac Galeni libri aliquot &c. Greek and Latin. 1532.
8° *539 a. 18 (1)* [B.M.]

—   Another edition. See Hippocrates. [Two or more works]
Hippocratis Aphorismi &c. 1539. 8° *539 a. 19 (2)* [B.M.]

—   Another edition. See Hippocrates [Two or more works]
Aphorismorum Hippocratis Sectiones septem &c. Greek and
Latin. 1543. 8° *539 a. 3* [B.M.]

—   Another edition. In Artem Medicinalem Galen, tabulæ et
commentarii : per T. Zuingerrum . . . (Galeni Ars Medicinalis
. . . Accessit . . . Index. Basileæ. 1561 fol. *539 k. 7 (2)* [B.M.]

—   Another edition. Galeni Ars Medicinalis argumentis . . .
locupletata e J. Thuilio. Patavii. 1622. 16° *544 a. 34 (2)*
[B.M.]

—   Another edition. Patavii. 1642. 12° *740 a. 17 (1)*
[B.M.]

—   Another edition. See Schola. Schola medica &c. 1647.
16° *549 a. 28* [B.M.]

—   Galeni Ars medicinalis per J. Manardum versa, divinis-q.
commentariolis adeo docte illustrata, ut clariss. Leonicenus,
omnes-q. alii superiores interpretes, insertiæ plane convicti
sint Romæ. 1525. 4° *540 e. 7 (1)* [B.M.]

—   Galeni Ars medicinalis. J. Manardo interprete. See
Psellus (M. C.) Pselli de victus ratione . . . libri II, &c.
1529. 8° *544 a. 3 (1)* [B.M.]

—   J. Manardi . . . in primum artis parvæ Galeni librum
comentaria, jam primum recens nata et ædita. Few MS. notes.
Basileæ. 1536. 4° *541 C. 13 (1)* [B.M.]

—   Claudii Galeni Ars medica quæ et Ars parva, M. Acakia
. . . interprete. Copious MS. notes. Parisiis, 1543. 4° *7320
f. 7* [B.M.]

— Another edition. Venetiis, 1544. 8° *540 d. 11* [B.M.]

— Another edition. Lugduni, 1548. 16° *774 a. 2* [B.M.]

— H. Thriveri in Τέχνην Galeni Commentarii (with Latin text). Lugduni, 1547. 12° *540 a. 21* [B.M.]

— Jacobi Foroliviensio . . . expositio et quæstiones in artem medicinalem Galeni quæ vulgo techni appellatur quam emendatissime (with the text in Latin). Venetiis, 1547 fol. *539 k. 8* [B.M.]

— J. Delphini . . . in III Galeno Artis Medicinalis Lib. explanatio. (With the Latin text.) Ejusdem de ratione medicamentorum præscribendorum liber. Lat. Venetiis, 1557. 4° *540 f. 5 (4)* [B.M.]

— In artem medicam Galeni commentarii, authore N. Biesio. (With the text in Latin, translated from the Greek by N. Biesius.) Antverpiæ, 1560. 8° *540 b. 24* [B.M.]

— Galeni Ars Medica, J.P. Ingrassia interprete, ac veluti novo plusquam commendatore. Venetiis, 1574 fol. *540 L. 14* [B.M.]

— Commentaria . . . in tres libros artis medicinalis Galeni auctore S. Sclano (with the text in Latin). Venetiis, 1597. 4° *540 g. 7* [B.M.]

— S. Sanctorii . . . commentaria in artem medicinalem Galeni . . . Multa in hac nova editione ab ipso auctore addita et emendata. (With the Latin text interpolated.) Venetiis, 1630. 4° *540 g. 8* [B.M.]

— Another edition. Lugduni, 1632. 4° *540 g. 9* [B.M.]

— J. Riolani . . . in artem parvam Galeni commentarius. (Edited by G. Nandæus. With the text.) Parisiis, 1631. 12° *974 a. 6 (1)* [B.M.]

— L. Tozzi . . . in librum artis medicinalis Galeni
παραφραστικὴ, ανακεφαλαίωσις &c.

Arranged in alternate paragraphs with the text in Latin. See Tozzi (L.) L. Tozzi . . . opera physico-medica &c. Tom. 5. 1703 &c. 4° *542 c. 14* [B.M.]

Ars medica—Greek and Latin

— Claudii Galeni liber . . . quem Τέχνην ἰατρικήν hoc est, artem medicinalem, inscripsit. Latinitate donatus partim a N. Leoniceno . . . partim a J. Manardo . . . Idem liber artis medicinalis . . . Græce additus . . . Commentarii . . . in eundem librii artis medicinalis . . . in lucem editi per J. A. Ammonium (Hippocratis de specie, acie, visuve, et opsios oculorum corrupta liber). Basileæ, 1541. 8° *540 b. 3* [B.M.]

— Ταληνοῦ τέχνη ἰατρική. Galeni Ars medicinalis, N. Leoniceno interprete. See Hippocrates. [Two or more works.] ῾Ιπποκρατους Κώου ᾽Αφορισμῶν βιβλ. Η', &c. Greek and Latin. 1543. 8° *539 b. 1* [B.M.]

— Artis parvæ Galeni caput octogesimum nonum, Greek and Latin. See PLANER (A.). A Planeri . . . de methodo medendi liber &c. 1583. 8° *544 b. 24* [B.M.]

Ard medica—Appendix

— See Angelucci (T.) Ars medica, ex Hippocratis, Galenique thesauris potissimum deprompta. 1588. 4° *539 f. 9 (1)* [B.M.]

— Fabii Paulini in libros artis medicinalis Galeni per tabulas œconomia. See Argenterius (J.) Opera &c. 1610 fol. *541 h. 5* [B.M.]

— See BÆRSDORP (C. A.) Methodus universæ artis medicæ formulis expressa ex Gal. traditionibus &c. 1538 fol. *1773 m. 4* [B.M.]

— See CITTADINI (A.) A. Cittadini . . . Auscultationes in Parvam artem Galeni. 1523 fol. *540 h. 9* [B.M.]

— See DU LAURENS (A.) Operum A. Laurentii . . . tomus alter. Continens . . . ejusdem annotationes in artem parvam Galeni &c. 1628 fol. *542 g. 13* [B.M.]

— See MONTANUS (J. B.) J. B. Montanii . . . in artem parvam Galeni explanationes &c. 1554. 8° *540 b. 27* [B.M.]

— 1556. 8° *540 a. 23* [B.M.]

— See Montanus (J. B.) Typus trium librorum artis parvæ Galeni &c. 1546 fol. *539 k. 9* [B.M.]

— Libellus introductorius in artem parvam Galeni de principiis universalibus totius medicinæ . . . ex doctrina Avicennæ . . . congestus.

— See MUHAMMAD IBN ZAKARIYA ABU BAKR. AL-RAZI &c. Opus . . . Galeatii de Sancta Sophia in nonu tractatum libri Rhasis ad regem Almansorem &c. 1533 fol. *543 g. 10 (1)* [B.M.]

— See ODDIS (O. De) O. de Oddis . . . Expositio in Librum artis Medicinalis Galeni &c. 1574. 4° *540 f. 9* [B.M.]

— See SEBISCH (M.) the Younger. Galeni ars parva in disputationes triginta resoluta. 1633 &c. 8° *1774 b. 13* [B.M.]

(9)

περὶ τῶν καθ᾽ Ἱπποκράτην στοιχείων

De elementis secumdum Hippocratem

Greek, Latin, and Arabic MSS. are known.

Latin MSS.

Avranches : nr. 232 ; s. xii/xiii, f. 126 et No. 9

Basle : Basil. D. III, 8 ; s. —

Breslau : Vratislav. Bibl. Univ. IV, F. 25 : s. xiii, f. 42

Cambridge : Cantabrig. St. Petri 33 ; s. xiii/xiv, f. 124 (" In tit. Galeno, in calce Hippocrati adscribitur ")

Chartres : Autricens. 284 (340) ; s. xiii, f. 1

Cues : Bibl. Nic. Cusani med. I ; s. xiii, No. 4

med. II ; s. xiii, No. 6

Dresden : Dresdens. Db. 91 ; s. xv, f. 1 (" Hippocratis liber de IV elementis ")

Eton : Bibl. Coll. 132 ; s. xiii, No. 15

Erfurt : Amplon. F. 249 ; s. xiii, f. 236

Leipzig : Lipsiens. bibl. univ. Repos. med I 4 ; s. —

I 22 ; s. —

1 29 ; s. — (sine auct. nomine ?)

Montpellier : Montepess. (École de méd.) 18 ; s. xiii

Munich : Monacens. 5 ; s. xiv, f. 1

                35 ; s. xiii, xiv, f. 55

Monast. Gaybæ. fol. 285 ; s. —

Oxford : Coll. Balliol 231 ; s. xiv in. f. 2

       B. Mariæ Magdal. 175 ; s. xiv, f. 172

       Merton, 218 ; s. xiv, f. 2

Paris : Parisin. 7015 ; s. xiv

           11860 ; s. xiv, f. 1

           14389 ; s. xiv, f. 1

           15456 ; s. xviii, f. 133

         nouv. acq. 343 ; s. xiii, f. 1

                1482 ; s. —, f. 78

Rome : Palat. 1094 ; s. xiv, f. 1

      Urbin.   235 ; s. xiv, f. 143

           247 ; s. xiv, f. 109

      Vatic. 2375 ; s. xiv, f. 91

         2381 ; s. —, f. 209

         3900 ; s. —, f. 45

Vendôme : Vindiocinens, 234 ; s. xiv, f. 54 (Expl. consistentes)

Latin translations

  — D. I, f. 25

  — C. I, f. 1 (Liber primus, Nicolao Leoniceno Interprete)

       f. 21 (Liber secundus, Nicolao Leoniceno Interprete)

  — Claudii Galeni de elementis libri duo, V. Trincavelio interprete. Adjecimus . . . Hippocratis librum de elementis (i.e. de natura humana, A. Brentio interprete) una cum commentario in eundem J. Sylvii (i.e. J. Du Bois). Lugduni, 1548. 8° *545 a. 1 (2)* [B.M.]

  — Another edition. Lugduni, 1558. 8° *545 a. 1 (3)* [B.M.]

  — Another copy. *540 a. 10 (2)* [B.M.]

De Elementis—Appendix

  — See Helmreich (G.). Observationes criticæ in Galeni de Elementis secundum Hippocratem libros. 1877. 8° *11312 h. 40 (4)* [B.M.]

(10)

περὶ κράσεων

De temperamentis

Greek, Arabic, and Latin MSS. are known.

Latin MSS.

Angers : Andecavens. 461 (446) ; s. xvi, f. 1 (Joh. Riolani
   annotatt. in libr. II de temperam : ætatum)

Basle : Basil. D.   I, 5 ; s. —

   D. III, 8 ; s —

Breslau : Vratisl. Bibl. Univ. IV, F. 25 ; s. xiii, f. 1

   IV, F. 26 ; s. —, f. 1

Cambridge : Cantabrig. St. Petri 33 ; s. xiii/xiv, f. 81b

Cesena : Malatest. D. XXV, 1 ; s. xiii, f. 29

   D. XXV, 2 ; s. xiii

   D. XXVI, 1 ; s. xiii

   S. V, 4 ; s. xiv, f. 102

   S. V, 5 ; s. xiv

Chartres : Autricens. 284 (340) ; s. xiii, f. 10

Cues : Bibl. Nic. Cusani med. II ; s. xiii, xiv, No. 4

Eton : Bibl. Coll. 132 ; s. xiii, No. 16

Erfurt : Amplon. F. 249 ; s. xiii, f. 213

   Q. 178* ; s. xiii, f. 158–9 (Libri abbreviati)

Hamburg : Offenbach. 105 ; s. —, f. 1

Leipzig : Lipsiens. bibl. univ. Repos. med. I, 4 ; s. —

   I, 29 ; s. — (sine
   auctoris nomine)

London : Addit. (Brit. Mus.) 22, 669 ; s. xiv, f. 28

   Harleian (Brit. Mus.) 3748 ; s. xv, f. 190

Munich : Monacens.   5 ; s. xiv, f. 127

   11 ; s. xiv, f. 96 (Initium tantum)

   35 ; s. xiii, xiv, f. 114 (mutil.)

   13054 (Rat. civ, 54) ; s. xiv, f. 174

Naples : Neapolit. VIII, D. 30 ; s. xiv
          Oratorian. 152 ; s. xiv–xv

Oxford : Oxon. Coll. Balliol, 213 ; s. xiv, in f. 263
          Merton, 218 ; s. xiv, f. 7b
               219 ; s. xiv in f. 17

Padua : Bibl. S. Joannis in Viridario, ad læv. plut. XVIII
        (Whereabouts not known)

Paris : Parisin.   7005 (?)
               7015 ; s. xiv, No. 3
               7026 ; s. xvi, No. 2 (Epitome)
             11860 ; s. xiv, f. 8
             14389 ; s. xiv, f. 11
             15455 ; s. xiii, f. 56
             16157 ; s. xiii, f. 1
          nouv. acq.   343 ; s. xiii, f. 14
                       1482 ; s. —, f. 58

Rome : Palat.   1092 ; s. —, f. 1
               1094 ; s. xiv, f. 11
               1095 ; s. xiv, f. 33
               1096 ; s. xiv, f. 1
       Urbin.   247 ; s. xiv, f. 69
       Vatic. 2375 ; s. xiv, f. 1
               2376 ; s. —, f. 1
               2378 ; s. —, f. 49
               2381 ; s. —, f. 116
               2383 ; s. —, f. 147
               2386 ; s. —, f. 31
               2389 ; s. —, f. 51
               2146* ; s. —, f. 56 [" Pars pænult. capitis
                  libri III Inc. incipiamus in hoc. Expl.
                  in medicinis ipsis "=Exit libri]

Latin translations

— D. I, f. 43

— C. I, f. 25 (Liber primus, Thoma Linacro Interprete)

  f. 43 (Liber secundus, Thoma Linacro Interprete)

  f. 63 (Liber tertius, Thoma Linacro Interprete)

— H. Thriveri . . . novi et integri commentarii in omnes Galeni libros de temperamentis. [With a translation of the text] H. Thriveri . . . in omnes Galeni de temperamentis libros epitome. 2 parts. Lugduni, 1547. 16° *540 a. 22 (1, 2)* [B.M.]

— E. Quercetani in libros Claudii Galeni de temperamentis Scholia. [With the text in Latin]

See Hippocrates. [De natura humana] Acroamaton in librum Hippocratis de natura hominis commentarius unus &c. 1549. 8° *539 b. 11* [B.M.]

— In libros Galeni de temperamentis novi et integri commentarii (with the text). G. Lopez Canario . . . autore. Compluti. 1565 fol. *540 h. 3 (2)* [B.M.]

Title page slightly mutilated.

— Claudii Galeni . . . aliquot opera L. Fuschio, Parisiis [1549–54] contains " De temperamentis libri tres ". *540 h. 2* [B.M.]

De temperamentis—Appendix

— See STUPANIS (J. N.) Claudii Galeni de temperamentis libri tres a J. N. Stupano contracti in propositiones &c. 1597. 4° *1179 g. 2 (4)* [B.M.]

(11)

περὶ φυσικῶν δυνάμεων

De facultatibus naturalibus

Greek, Arabic, and Latin MSS. are known.

Latin MSS.

  Angers : Andecavens. 461 (446) ; s. xvi, f. 11 (Jo. Riolani annotatt.)

Basle : Basil. D. III, 8 : s. —

Bourges : Biturigens. 299 (247) ; s. xiv, f. 1

Cambridge : Cantabrig. [Caius Coll. 947 ; s. —]
     St. Petri 33 ; s. xiii/xiv, f. 69b

Cesena : Malatest. D. XXV, 1 ; s. xiii f. 11
        S. XXVII, 4 ; s. xiv, No. 8 (Anon. Comm.)

Chartres : Autricens. 293 (351) ; s. xiv, f. 105

Erfurt : Amplon. F. 249 ; s. xiii, f. 195

Florence : Laurent. plut. 73, 11 ; s. xiv, f. 57

Heidelberg : Bibl. Univ. 1080* ; s. xiii, xiv, No. 13

Leipzig : Lipsiens. bibl. univ. Repos. med. I, 4 ; s. —
             II, 49 ; s. —
             (Lectt. in Gal.
             lib.)

Montecassino : Casinens. 70 ; s. xiv, p. 147 ; (Expl. mutil. ;
        ambo vera hoc et prædicta)

Montpellier : Montepess. (École de Méd.) 18 ; s. xiii

Munich : Monacens.   5 ; s. xiv, f. 203
       35 ; s. xiii, xiv, f. 99
     13054 (Rat. civ, 54) ; s. xiv, f. 178 (Nic.
         Bononiens expos.)

Oxford : Oxon. Coll. Balliol 231 ; s. xiv, in f. 10
     Caii. 947 ; s. —

Paris : Parisin. 11860 ; s. xiv, f. 149
     14389 ; s. xiv, f. 34
     15456 ; s. xiii, f. 3

Rome : Palat. 1094 ; s. xiv, f. 410
     1095 ; s. xiv, f. 69
     1096 ; s. xiv, f. 128
   Urbin. 247 ; s. xiv, f. 137

Vatic. 2375 ; s. xiv, f. 401

2376 ; s. —, f. 171

2378 ; s. —, f. 212

2383 ; s. —, f. 1

2384 ; s. —, f. 1

2386 ; s. —, f. 69

2389 ; s. —, f. 66

4432 ; s. —, f. 102–4 (Expl. mutil. : vocantur hinc . . .)

Venice : Marcian. cl. XIV, 5 ; s. xiv, f. 13

Volterra : Volaterran. 103 (6365) ; s. xv, f. 65

Latin translations

— D. I, f. 103

— C. I, f. 905 to 964 (Libri III Thoma Linacro anglo Interprete)

— Galeni de naturalib. facultatibus libri tres, T. Linacro . . . interprete. Antverpiæ, 1547. 8° *540 b. 4 (1)* [B.M.]

— Galeni . . . de naturalibus facultatibus libri tres . . . T. Linacro . . . interprete. (Edited by J. Guinterius.) Few MS. notes. Paris, 1528. 8° *540 b. 13 (1)* [B.M.]

De Naturalibus Facultatibus—Appendix

— See COSCHWICHIUS (J.) *Resp.* Disputatio de naturalibus facultatibus sexta ex capitibus 6–9 libri secundi Galeni de naturalibus facultatibus. 1645. 4° *1179 i. 6 (6)* [B.M.]

— See FREY (J.) Disputatio de naturalibus facultatibus quarta ; ex capitibus 12–17 libri primi Galeni de naturalibus facultatibus &c. 1645. 4° *1179 i. 5 (28)* [B.M.]

— See HARDERUS (C.) Disputatio de naturalibus facultatibus prima ; continens trium librorum Galeni de naturalibus facultatibus argumentum &c. 1644. 4° *1179 i. 5 (25)* [B.M.]

— See SEBISCH (M.) the Younger. Disputatio de naturalibus facultatibus prima (—secunda) ; continens trium librorum

Galeni de Naturalibus Facultatibus argumentum &c. 1644 &c.
4° *1179 i. 6 (1, 2)* [B.M.]

An English translation of this work together with the Greek
text has recently been issued in the Loeb Classical Series. This
is the only Galenic writing that has been published in English.

(12)

περὶ ἀνατομικῶν ἐγχειρήσεων

De anatomicis administrationibus

This Galenic work is of peculiar interest. The first nine
books are known in the Greek manuscript (at Copenhagen,
Florence, Leipzig, Leyden, Milan, Modena, Oxford, Padua, Paris,
and Venice). Books x–xv are in the Arabic MSS. (see Ch. II),
while a Latin translation, together with the English by the late
Dr. Greenhill, is at the Royal College of Physicians (Schedæ
Greenhill). More recently, Max Simon has published a German
translation with full *apparatus criticus* of books x–xv.

Latin translations

— C. I, f. 185 (Libri nouem, ab Johanne Andernaco Latinate
donati, and nuper ab Andrea Vesalio Brusellensi correcti, ac
pene alii facti)

> f. 203 (Liber Secundus)
> f. 219 (Liber Tertius)
> f. 239 (Liber Quartus)
> f. 255 (Liber Quintus)
> f. 271 (Liber Sextus)
> f. 287 (Liber Septimus)
> f. 303 (Liber Octauus)
> f. 319 (Liber Nonus)

— Claudii Galeni . . . de anatomicis administrationibus,
libri IX. Joannem (Guinterio) Andernaco interprete. Lugduni,
1551. 8° *540 a. 11* [B.M.]

— Oribasii anatomica ex libris Galeni, cum versione Latina
J. B. Rasarii, curante G. Dundass, cujus notæ accedunt. Greek
and Latin. Lugduni Batavorum, 1735. 4° *541 e. 17* [B.M.]

(13)

περὶ ὀστῶν τοῖς εἰσαγομένοις

De ossibus ad Tirones

Greek, Latin, and Arabic MSS. are known.

Latin MSS.

Paris : Parisin (6816 [? Comm. anon.]) 6878 ; s. xvi, No. 1
(Anon. comm. in Gal. de ossibus)

Latin translations

— C. I, f. 143 (Inscr. Cl. Galeni de Ossibus ad Tyrones
Liber, Ferdinando Balamio Siculo Interprete)

De ossibus &c.—Greek and Latin

— J. P. Ingrassiæ . . . in Galeni librum de ossibus . . .
commentaria . . . Quibus appositus est Græcus Galeni con-
textus, una cum . . . ajusdem Ingrassiæ in Latinum versione.
Greek and Latin. Panormi. 1603 fol. *540 h. 15 (1)* [B.M.]

— Γαληνοῦ περὶ ὀστῶν. Claudii Galeni . . . de ossibus ad
tyrones liber, F. Balamio interprete. Cum notis . . . C.
Hofmanni &c. Francofurti ad Mænum. 1630 fol. *778 i. 4 (3)*
[B.M.]

— Galenus de ossibus Græce et Latine. Accedunt Vesalii,
Sylvii, Heneri, Eustachii ad Galeni doctrinam exercitationes.
(Hippocrates de ossium natura. A. C. Celsus de positu et figura
ossium totius humani corporis.) Ex Bibliotheca J. Van. Horne.
Lugduni Batavorum, 1665. 12° *540 b. 11* [B.M.]

De ossibus &c.—Latin

— Galenus de ossibus. F. Balamio . . . interprete ad
Græcorum codicum fidem . . . emendatus, et scholiis illustratus.
Latin. Lyons, 1549. 8° *540 a. 5 (1)* [B.M.]

— Another edition. Enarrationibus illustratus a L. Collado Valentino &c. Valentiæ, 1555. 8° *7421 a. 31* [B.M.]

— Another edition. Copious MS. notes. Rostochii, 1636. 8° *540 b. 15 (4)* [B.M.]

— Liber Galeni de ossibus. See RIOLAN (J.) the Younger. Osteologia &c. 1614. 8° *548 c. 5* [B.M.]

De ossibus ad Tirones—Appendix

— See FALLOPPIO (G.). G. Falloppii . . . Expositio in librum Galeni de ossibus &c. 1570. 4° *546 g. 4 (2)* [B.M.]

(14)
περὶ φλεβῶν καὶ ἀρτηριῶν ἀνατομῆς
De venarum arteriarumque dissectione

Of the MSS. only the Greek and Arabic survive. The Latin MSS. are lost.

Latin translations

— C. I, f. 161 (Inscr. Cl. Galeni De venarum arteriarumque dissectione Liber, Ab Antonio Fortolo Ioseriensi Latinate donatus, & ab Andrea Vuesalio Bruxellensi plerisque in locis recognitus)

— Dissectione venarum arteriarumque commentarium. Ejusdem de nervis compendium A. Fortolo interprete. Let. Basileæ. 1529. 18° *547 a. 3* [B.M.]

(15)
περὶ νεύρον ἀνατομῆς
De nervorum dissectione

Of the MSS. only the Greek and Arabic are known.

Latin translations

— C. I, f. 157 (Inscr. Cl. Galeni De nervorum dissectione Liber, Ab Antonio Fortolo Ioseriensi Latinate donatus, & ab Andrea Vuesalio Bruxellensi aliquot in locis recognitus)

— Dissectionis venarum arteriarumque commentarium. Ejusdem de nervis compendium A. Fortolo interprete. Let. Basileæ. 1529. 18° *547 a. 3* [B.M.]

(16)

περὶ ὀσφρήσεως ὀργάνου

De instrumento odoratus

Of the MSS. only the Greek are known.

Latin translations

— C. I, f. 331 (Inscr. Cl. Galeni De instrumento odoratus, Ludouico Bellisario Medico Mutinensi Interprete)

(17)

περὶ μήτρας ἀνατομῆς

De uteri dissectione

Greek MSS. survive.

Latin translations

— D. I, f. 60

— C. I, f. 325 (Inscr. Cl. Galeni De dissectione Vulvæ Libellus, Joanne Bernardo Feliciano Interprete)

— De uteri dissectione. [Translated by J. Cornarius] See Marcellus, Empiricus. Marcelli de medicamentis empiricis liber &c. 1531 fol. *539 k. 16 (1–5)* [B.M.]

— In Hippocratem Commentarii

(18)

περὶ χρείας τῶν ἐν ἀνθρώπου σώματι μορίων λόγοι ιζ′

De usu partium corporis humani libri XVII

Greek and Latin MSS. of the seventeen books are known.

Latin MSS.

Dresden : Dresd. Db. 92, 93 ; s. xv, f. 54c

Madrid : Martit. bibl. nac. 1196 (ol. L. 9)* ; s. xiv, f. 160 et 164

Munich : Monacens, 26 ; s. xv

Rome : Vatic. 2380 ; s. xv, f. 1

Latin translations

— D. II, f. 209

— C. I, f. 341 (Inscr. Cl. Galeni De usu partium corporis
libri septendecim, Nicolao Regio Calabro Interprete, Denuo
extractiori cura ad Græci exemplaris veritatem castigati per
Jacobum Sylvium Medicum, & Martinum Gregorium)

— Claudii Galeni Pergameni, secundum Hippocratem . . .
opus de usu partium corporis humanio magna cura ad exemp, aris
Græci veritatem castigatum . . . Nicolao Regio . . . interprete.
MS. notes. Ex officina Simonis Colinæi : Parisiis, 1528. 4°
540 g. 5 [B.M.]

— Another edition. Lugduni, 1550. 8° *540 a. 9* [B.M.]

— Erotemata in Galeni de usu partium in hominis corpore,
libros XVII. [With part of the text.] Per J. Leonicenum.
Franc. [ofurti] 1550. 8° *540 b. 15 (1)* [B.M.]

— Augustæ Laudes Divinæ Majestatis . . . a centum
undequadraginta miraculis in homine e . . . Galeni de usu
partium libris XVII selectæ . . . dilucidis explenationibus
illustratæ . . . ab S. Meyero &c. Friburgi Brisgoriæ. 1627.
12° *1121 C. 35* [B.M.]

De usu partium corporis humani—Appendix

See HOFMANNUS (C.) C. Hofmanni commentarii in Galeni de
usu partium corporis humani lib. XVII &c. 1625 fol. *539 k. 14*
[B.M.]

— See Theophilus, Protospatharius. Theophili Protospatarii
in Galeni de usu partium libros epitome, quam de corporis
humani fabrica inscripsit. 1540. 12° *540 a. 4 (1)* [B.M.]

De iuvamentis membrorum libri X

This work consists of a portion of the " De usu partium
corporis humani libri XVII ", and is known in Arabic and
Latin manuscript.

" Libri De iuvamentis partium, compendia sunt librorum De usu partium " (See Gal. Op., ed. Lugduni, 1550, to 5—Elenchus librorum Galeni omnium qui in hoc opere continentur)

Latin MSS.

Breslau : Vratislav. bibl. univ. IV, F. 25* ; s. xiii, f. 68–91 (Ex IX libris prioribus)

Cambridge : Cantabr. St. Petri 33 ; s. xiii/xiv, f. 222b

Cesena : Malatest. D. XXV, 2 ; s. xiii
S. XXVII, 4 ; s. xiv, No. 1

Chartres : Autricens. 284 (340) ; s. xiii, f. 64

Cues : Bibl. Nic. Cusani med. I ; s. xiii, No. 3
II ; s. xiii, xiv, No. 3

Eton : Bibl. Coll. 132 ; s. xiii, No. 14

Erfurt : Amplon. F. 249; s. xiii, f. 259 (Libri IX. Expl. anatomicos vocare eas)

London : Addit. (Br. Mus.) 22, 669 ; s. xiv, f. 49
Harleian. 3748 ; s. xv, f. 168 (Libri IX. Corresponds to Amplon)

Montpellier : Montepess. (École de Méd.) 18 ; s. xiii

Munich : Monac. 5 ; s. xiv, f. 221 (Liber de iuvamentis membrorum recollectus a libro Galeni de utilitate particularum)

Oxford : Coll. Balliol 231 ; s. xiv in f. 56b (Libri IX. Expl. anatomicos notantes eas. Vide Amplon.)

Paris : Bibl. de l'Arsenal 1080* ; s. xiv, f. 25
Parisin. 11860 ; s. xiv, f. 22
14389 ; s. xiv, f. 54
15455 ; s. xiii, f. 72

Perugia : Perusin. 44 (A. 44); s. xv, f. 45–51 (Inc. Et patet quod dicit)

Rome : Palat.   1094 ; s. xiv, f. 88
              1099 ; s. xv, f. 1 (libri IX)
       Urbin.   247 ; s. xiv, f. 88
       Vatic.   2375 ; s. xiv, f. 215
              2376 ; s. —, f. 119
              2378 ; s. —, f. 63
              2382 ; s. —, f. 37
              2383 ; s. —, f. 51
              2386 ; s. —, f. 51
              2389 ; s. —, f. 3

Subiaco : nr. 59 ; s. xiii, f. 63

Latin translations

— D. I, f. 61 (Inc. Corpora animalium sunt instrumenta
Expl. tamen inter suturas nominantur)

(19)

περὶ μυῶν κινήσεως βιβλ. β'

De motu musculorum libri II

Greek and Latin MSS. are known.

A *Latin MS.* is Basil. D. III, 8 ; s. — (De motu membrorum
seu de motu musculorum)

Latin translations

— C. I, f. 965 (Lib. I.   Inscr. Claudii Galeni De motu muscu-
lorum, liber primus, Thoma Linacro Anglo Interprete ; lib. II
inscr. Claudii Galeni De motu musculorum, liber secundus,
Nicolao Leoniceno Interprete)
— Claudii Galeni . . . de motu musculorum libri duo.
N. Leoniceno interprete . . . libellus . . . castigatus, et . . .
scholiis illustratus per J. Syl. [vium., i.e. J. Du Bois.]
Lugduni. 1549.   8° *540 a. 4 (3)* [B.M.]

(20)

περὶ τῶν τῆς ἀναπνοῆς αἰτίων

De causis respirationis

Greek and Latin MSS. are known.

Latin MSS.

Cesena : Malatest. S. V, 4 ; s. xiv, f. 29

Chartres : Autricens. 293 (351) ; s. xiv, f. 118

Dresden : Dresd. Db. 92, 93 ; s. xv, f. 20a

Erfurt : Amplon. f. 236 ; s. xiv

Madrid : Matrit. 1978 (ol. L. 60) ; s. xiv, f. 93

Paris : Parisin. 6865 ; s. xiv, f. 124a

          7015 ; s. xiv

Rome : Palat. 1089 ; s. —, f. 114

      Vatic. 2378 ; s. —

Latin translations

— D. I, f. 84

— C. I, f. 713 (Jano Cornario Medici Interprete)

— De causis respirationis [Translated by J. Cornarius]

See Marcellus, Empiricus. Marcelli de medicamentis empiricis liber &c. 1531 fol. *539 k. 16 (1–5)* [B.M.]

(21)

περὶ χρείας ἀναπνοῆς

De respirationis usu

Greek and Latin MSS. are known.

Latin MSS.

Cesena : Malatest. S V 4 ; s. iv, f. 29

Chartres : Autricens. 293 (351) ; s. xiv, f. 116

Dresden : Dresd. Db 92, 93 ; s. xv, f. 20b

Erfurt : Amplon. F 77a ; s. xiv–xv, f. 108 (Expl. species monor simul.)

Paris : Parisin. 6865 ; s. xiv, f. 67b

Latin translations

— D. I, f. 84

— C. I, f. 701 (Inscr. Cl. Galeni De utilitate respirationis, liber unus, Jano Cornario Medico Interprete). The index of tome 1, however, refers to this work as De usu respirationis.

(22)

περὶ σπέρματος βιβλ. β'

De semine libri II

Known in the Greek and Latin MSS.

Latin MSS.

    Basle : Basil. D III 8 ; s. —

    Dresden : Dresd. Db 92, 93 ; s. xv, f. 43

    Paris : Parisin. 6865 ; s. xiv, f. 57

    Rome : Vatic. 2384 ; s. —, f. 79

Latin translations

— D. I, f. 31

— C. I, f. 1031 (Libro duo, Joanne Bernardo Feliciano interprete)

— De Semine libri II. [Translated by J. Cornarius.] See Marcellus, Empiricus. Marcelli de medicamentis empiricis liber &c. 1531 fol. *539 k. 16 (1–5)* [B.M.]

— Claudii Galeni Pergameni libro duo de semine, J. Guinterio Andernaco interprete. Adjectæ sunt ad calcem Græci exemplaris castigationes aliquot. Few MS. notes. Apud Simonem Colinæum Parisiis. 1533. 8° *1173 g. 12* [B.M.]

De semine—Appendix

— See FRANZOSIUS (H.) H. Franzosii Tractatus apologicus de Semine pro Aristotele adversus Galenum. 1645. 4° *778 f. 9* [B.M.]

(23)

περὶ κυουμένων διαπλάσεως

De fœtum formatione

Greek and Latin MSS. are known.

A *Latin MS.* is Dresd. Db 92, 93 ; s. xv, f. 295c (De formatione fœtus)

Latin translations

— D. I, f. 41 (Nicolao de Regio interprete)
— C. I, f. 1009 (Joanne Bernardo de Feliciani interprete)
— De fœtus formatione. [Translated by J. Cornarius.]
See MARCELLUS, Empiricis. Marcelli de medicamentis empiricis liber &c. 1531 fol. *539 k. 16 (1–5)* [B.M.]

(24)

εἰ κατὰ φύσιν ἐν ἀρτηρίαις αἷμα περιέχεται

An in arteriis natura sanguinis contineatur

Of the MSS. only the Greek survive (at Florence and Venice).

Latin translations

— C. I, f. 175 (Inscr. Galeni an in santuinis in arteriis natura contineatur, Jul. Martiano Rota Interprete)

(25)

περὶ ἀρίστης κατασκευῆς τοῦ σώματος ἡμῶν

De optima corporis nostri constitutione

Greek, Arabic, and Latin MSS. are known.

Latin MSS.

Cesena : Malatest. S V 4 ; s. xiv, f. 37
             S XXVI 4 ; s. xiii, f. 26 et 123
Chartres : Autricens. 293 (351) ; s. xiv, f. 125
London : Addit. (Br. Mus.) 22, 669 ; s. xiv, f. 47

Munich : Monacens.   5 ; s. xiv, f. 181
                    490 ; a. 1488–1503

Paris : Parisin. 6865 ; s. xiv, f. 79a

Rome : Vatic. 2378 ; s. —
              2417 ; s. —, f. 256

Latin translations

— D. I, f. 56

— C. I, f. 137 (Ferdinando Balamio Siculo Interprete)

(26)

περὶ εὐεξίας

De bono habitu

Greek, Arabic, and Latin MSS. are known.

Latin MSS.

Cesena : Malatest. S V 4 ; s. xiv, f. 38
                     S XXVI 4 ; s. xiii, f. 26 and after f. 123

Chartres : Autricens. 293 (351) ; s. xiv, f. 125

London : Addit. (Br. Mus.) 22, 669 ; s. xiv, after f. 47

Munich : Monac.   5 ; s. xiv, after f. 181
                  490 ; a. 1488–1503

Paris : Parisin. 6865 ; s. xiv, f. 80a

Rome : Palat. 1098 ; s. xv, f. 16
       Vatic. 2378 ; s. —, f. 243

Latin translations

— D. I, f. 56

— C. I, f. 141 (Inscr. Claudii Galeni De bona habitudine Liber. Ferdinando Balamio Siculo Interprete)

— De bono corporis habitu. See Blemmidas (N.) G. Valla . . . interprete. Hoc in volumine hec continentur ; Nicephori logica &c. 1498 fol. *8461 f. 6* [B.M.]

(27)

περὶ οὐσίας τῶν φυσικῶν δυνάμεων

De substantia facultatum naturalium fragmentum

Greek- Arabic- and Latin MSS. are known.

Latin MSS.

Cesena : Malatest. S V 4 ; s. xiv, f. 26

S XXVI 4 ; s. xiii, f. 14

Madrid : Matrit. bibl. nac. 1978 (ol. L 60) ; s. xiv, f. 101

Munich : Monacens. 490 ; a. 1488–1503

Paris : Parisin. 6865 ; s. xiv, f. 117c

Latin translations

— D. I, f. 103

— C. I, f. 723 (Bartholomæo Sylvanio Salonensi Interprete)

(28)

ὅτι τὰ τῆς ψυχῆς ἤθη ταῖς τοῦ σώματος κράσεσιν ἕπεται

Quod animi mores corporis temperamenta sequantur

Greek and Latin MSS. are known.

A *Latin MS.* is Dred. Db 92, 93 ; s. xv, f. 304d

Latin translations

— D. I, f. 115 (Nicolao de Regio interprete)

— C. I, f. 993 (Bartholomæo Sylvanio Salonensi interprete)

— J. B. Personæ . . . in Galeni lib. cui titulus est Quod animi mores corporis temperiem. sequuntur commentarius singularis. Bergomi 1602. 4° *540 f. 10* [B.M.]

— Iwani Muelleri specimen novæ editionis libri Galeniani qui inscribitur ʽοτι ταῖς τοῦ σώματος κεάσεσιν αἰτῆς ψυχῆς δυνάμεις ἕπονται. (Specimen alterum &c.) 2 parts. Erlangæ. 1880–5. 4° *7305 f. 2 (2)* [B.M.]

(29)

περὶ διαγνώσεως καὶ θεραπείας τῶν ἐν τῇ ἑκάστου ψυχῇ
ἰδίων παθῶν

De propriorum animi cuiuslibet affectuum dignotione et curatione

Greek and Latin MSS. are known.   A *Latin MS.* is Dresd. Db
92, 93 ; s. xv, f. 17 (Liber de cognitione propriorum defectuum et
viciorum translatus ab Armengando Blazii de Arabicio in
Latinum in Monte Pessulano. Inc. Quesivisti a me ut copularem.
Expl. longo tempore absque ratione).   The Arabic original is lost.

(30)

περὶ διαγνώσεως καὶ θεραπείας τῶν ἐν τῇ ἑκάστου ψυχῇ
ἰδίων ἁμαρτημάτων

De cuiuslibet animi peccatorum dignotione atque medela

The Greek MSS. are known.

Latin translations

—   C. I, f. 1244 (Inscr. Claud. Galeni De cuiusque animi
peccatorum notitia atque medela Libellus Junio Paulo Crasso
Patauino Interprete)

—   De viciis animi et eorum remediis.   See C. Galeni aliquot
oibelli &c.   1529.   4°   *540 f. 3* [B.M.]

(31)

περὶ μελαίνης χόλης

De atra bile

A number of Greek MSS. survive, while a single Latin MS.
Petropol. Firk. 332, 26, which is a translation by Stephen from
the Arabic of Hunayn, is mentioned by Steinschneider (Die
Hebräischen Uebersetzungen des Mittelalters, Berlin, 1893,
p. 655).   This MS. is entitled *De melancholia.*

Latin translations

—   C. I, f. 125 (Bartholomæo Sylvanio Salonensi Interprete)

— C. IV, f. 1183 (Inscr. De melancholia ex Galeno Rufo,
& Posidonio ab Ætio conscripta. Jano Cornario medico Interprete)

— De melancholia sive atræ bilis morbo ex Galeni, Rufi
et Ætii Sicamii voluminibus . . . collectanea una cum Stephani
Medici cognomento Magistri . . . oculari collyrio nunc primum
Latine ædita. M. T. Melanelio . . . interprete. 9 ff. Antverpiæ,
1540. 4° *540 e. 11 (2)* [B.M.]

— Another copy. *1191 k. 1 (1)* [B.M.]

(32)

περὶ χρείας σφυγμῶν

De usu pulsuum

Greek and Latin MSS. survive.

Latin MSS.

Basle : Basil. D III 8 ; s. —
Bourges : Biturgens. 299 (247) ; s. xiv, f. 137
Cambridge : Cantabr. Caius Coll. 948 ; s. —
Cesena : Malatest. D. XXV. 2 ; s. xiii (Inscr. De pulsu)
           S V 4 ; xiv, f. 56
Chartres : Autricens. 284 (340) ; s. xiii, f. 132
Dresden : Dresd. Db 92, 93 ; s. xv, f. 39b
Erfurt : Amplon. F 249 : s. xiii, f. 185
           F 276 ; s. xiv, f. 69
Leipzig : Lipsiens. bibl. univ. Repos. med. I 4 ; s. —
Montecassino : Casinens. 70 ; s. xiv, p. 148
Moulins : nr. 30 ; s. xiv, f. 90
Oxford : Coll. Balliol, 231 ; s. xiv, in. f. 48b
Paris : Parisin. 7011 (?) ; s. xvi
           7015 ; s. xiv
         11860 ; s. xiv, f. 225
         15455 ; s. xiii, f. 162

Rome : Palat.   1094 ; s. xiv, f. 202 et 547
 Urbin.   247 ; s. xiv, f. 117
 Vatic.   2376 ; s. —, f. 91
 2378 ; s. —, f. 94
 2383 ; s. —, f. 142
Venice : Marcian. cl. XIV, 6 ; s. xiv, f. 54

Latin translations

— D. I, f. 87 (Marco Toletano interprete)

— D. I, f. 715 (Thoma Linacro Anglo Interprete)

— Galenus Pergamenus de pulsuum usu, T. Linacro interprete. Few MS. notes. In ædibus Pinsonianis, Londini. 1522 4° *540 e. 6 (1)* [B.M.]

Eighteen leaves without pagination.

(33)

περὶ τῶν ῾Ιπποκράτους καὶ Πλάτωνος δογμάτων βιβλία θ'

De placitis Hippocratis et Platonis libri IX

The Greek MSS. are known.

Latin translations

— C. I, f. 727 (Inscr. Cl. Galeni De decretis Hippocratis & Platonis Liber Primus, sine principio, Joanne Caio Britanno Interprete). Libri II–IX. Joanne Bernardo Feliciano Interprete.

— Claudii Galeni de placitis Hippocratis et Platonis libri novem. Recensuit et explanavit Iwanus Mueller. Greek and Latin. Tom. 1. No more published. Lipsiæ, 1874. 8° *7305 c. 10* [B.M.]

— Claudii Galeni de Hippocratis et Platonis Dogmatibus libri IX. J. Cornario interprete. Lugduni, 1550. 12° *540 a. 8* [B.M.]

— See KALBFLEISCH (C.). In Galeni de placitis Hippocratis et Platonis libros observationes criticæ. 1892. 8° *11312 p. 17 (3)* [B.M.]

— See Petersen (J.) Dr. Phil. In Galeni de placitis Hippocratis et Platonis libros quæstiones criticæ. 1888. 8° *11312
m. 23 (4)* [B.M.]

(34)

Θρασύβουλος, πότερον ἰατρικῆς ἢ γυμναστικῆς ἐστι τὸ ὑγιεινόι
Thrasybulus sive utrum medicinæ sit an gymnastices hygieine
The Greek MSS. survive.

(35)

περὶ τοῦ διὰ τῆς σμικρᾶς σφαίρας γυμνασίου
De parvæ pilæ exercitio
Greek and Latin MSS. survive.

Latin MSS.

Cesena : Malatest. S V 4 ; s. xiv, f. 36
        S XXVI 4 ; s. xiii, f. 23
Munich : Monacens. 490 ; a. 1488–1503
Oxford : Oxon. Coll. Omn. Animar. 68 ; s. xiv, f. 189
Paris : Parisin. 6865 ; s. xiv, f. 74b
Rome : Palat. 1098 ; s. xv, f. 5
        Vatic. 2378 ; s. —, f. 244
               2384 ; s. —, f. 28

Latin translations

— D. I, f. 144
— C. I, f. 1220 (Valerio Centannio Vicentino Interprete)
— Claudii Gal. de exercitatione, quæ pila suscipitur, commentarius, Jacobo Gupulo Pictavo interprete. Parisiis. 1544.
8° *774 b. 30 (4)* [B.M.]
— Claudius Galenus de parvæ pilæ exercitio, J. Cornario
interprete. See Polybus. Polybi de diæta salubri . . . libellus
&c. 1561. 12° *774 a. 18* [B.M.]

(36)

περὶ ἀφροδισίων

De venereis

A single Greek MS. is known.

(37)

'Υγιεινῶν λόγοι ζ'

De sanitate tuenda libri VI

Greek, Arabic, and Latin MSS. are known.

Latin MSS.

Angers : Andecavens. 461 (446)* ; s. xvi, f. 217 (Passarti
            annotatt.)

Basle : Basil. D I, 5 ; s. —

Berne : Berens. 80 ; s. xv, f. 82

Bourges : Biturigens. 299 (247) ; s. xiv, f. 150

Breslau : Vratislav. bibl. univ. IV F 25* ; s. xiii, f. 56–8
            (Exc. e libr. I–V et integ. conversus I, VI)

Cambridge : Cantabr. St. Petri 33 ; s. xiii/xiv, f. 207b

Cesena : Malatest. D XXIII 1 ; s. xiii
            S XXVII 4 ; s. xiv, No. 9 (Anon. Comm.)

Cues : Bibl. Nic. Cusani med. 11 ; s. xiii, xiv, No. 9

Erfurt : Amplon. F 249 ; s. xiii, f. 109
            F 278 ; s. xiv in f. 29

Florence : Laurent. plut. 73, 11 ; s. xiv, f. 33

Leipzig : Lipsiens. bibl. univ. Repos. med. I 22 ; s. —

Madrid : Matrit. bibl. nac. 1198 (ol. L 9) ; s. xiv, f. 148 (L. VI
            init. mutil.)

Montpellier : Montepess. (École de méd.) 18 ; s. xiii

Munich : Monacens. 5 ; s. xiv, f. 42, 11 ; s. xiv, f. 45
                      35 ; s. xiii, xiv, f. 2

Oxford : Coll. Balliol. 231 ; s. xiv, in f. 216

Paris : Parisin. 6865A ; s. xiv

              6867 ; s. xv

           15456 ; s. xiii, f. 115

Rome : Palat. 1093 ; s. xiv, f. 112

             1094 ; s. xiv, f. 461

             1095 ; s. xiv, f. 54

             1096 ; s. xiv, f. 66

             1098 ; s. xv, f. 33

     Urbin.   247 ; s. xiv, f. 21

     Vatic. 2369 ; s. —, f. 60

             2375 ; s. xiv, f. 479

             2376 ; s. —, f. 20

             2382 ; s. —, f. 15

             2384 ; s. —, f. 14

             2385 ; s. —, f. 168

             4561 ; s. — (Gal. de virtutibus et bono regimine Juda filio Salomonis interpr. Inc. Sivas quod societas)

Venice : Marcian. cl. XIV 5 ; s. xiv, f. 1

                   6 ; s. xiv, f. 9

Latin translations

  — D. I, f. 225 (Burgundione Pisano interprete)

  — C. II, f. 5 (libri sex, Thoma Linacro interprete, recogniti)

  — Galeni de sanitate tuenda libri sex, T. Linacro Anglo interprete. [With dedication to Cardinal Wolsey, by T. Linacre in MS.] On vellum. Per G. Rubeum : Parisiis. 1517 fol. *C. 19 e. 15* [B.M.]

  — Another edition. Venetiis, 1523. 4° *540 e. 6 (2)* [B.M.]

  — Another edition. Colonie, 1526. 8° *540 d. 4* [B.M.]

  — Another edition. Parisiis, 1538. 8° *540 d. 5 (1)* [B.M.]

  — Another copy. Few MS. notes. *540 d. 6 (1)* [B.M.]

  — Another edition. Claudii Galeni . . . de sanitate tuenda libri sex, et nunc recens annotationibus a L. Fuchsio . . .

illustrati. 2 parts. Few MS. notes. Tubingæ, 1541. 8° *540 d. 8* [B.M.]

— Another edition. MS. notes. Lugduni, 1549. 8° *774 a. 3* [B.M.]

De Sanitate Tuenda—*Appendix*

— See BORDINGUS (J.) J. Bordingi enarrationes quæ commentariorum vice esse possunt in VI libros Galeni de sanitate tuenda &c. 1605. 8° *774 b. 12* [B.M.]

(38)

περὶ τροφῶν δυνάμεως βιβλία γ′

De alimentorum facultatibus libri III

Greek, Syriac, Arabic, and Latin MSS. are known.

Latin MSS.

Breslau : Vratisl. bibl. univ. IV F 25 ; s. xiii, f. 141–57
Cesena : D XXIII 1 ; s. xiii
        D XXV 1 ; s. xiii, f. 1
Florence : Laurent. plut. 73, 11 ; s. xiv, f. 1
Glasgow : Hunterian. U 4. 7 ; s. xiv, f. 1
Munich : Monacens. 5 ; s. xiv, f. 183
           35 ; s. viii, xiv, f. 38
Oxford : Coll. Balliol. 231 ; s. xiv in f. 233b
      Merton, 685 ; s. —
Paris : Parisin. 6865 ; s. xiv, f. 93b
Rome : Palat. 1094 ; s. xiv, f. 572
      Urbin. 247 ; s. xiv, f. 1
      Vatic. 2375 ; s. xiv, f. 423
          2376 ; s. —, f. 145
          2378 ; s. —, f. 43
          2382 ; s. —, f. 65
          2385 ; s. —, f. 137
          2386 ; s. —, f. 121

Venice : Marcian. 317 ; s. xiv

   App. cl. XIV 5 ; s. xiv, f. 25

The following are MSS. of this work inscribed *De cibis* or
De virtutibus cibariorum or similar titles.

Basle : Basil. D I 5 ; s. — (Libell. de alimentis e leguminibus
   percip. et aliis plantis . . . et Libell. de aliment.
   ex eximalibus)

Bourges : Biturigens. 299 (247) ; s. xiv, f. 50

Breslau : Vratisl. bibl. univ. IV F 25 ; s. xiii, f. 166–8 (De
   virtutibus alimentorum)

Cues : Bibl. Nic. Cusani med. 1 ; s. xiii, No. 2 (De virtutibus
   ciborum) et No. 6 (De cibis et potu)

   Bibl. Nic. Cusani med. 8 ; s. xiii, No. 3 (Inscribed the
   same as Cusani No. 2)

   Bibl. Nic. Cusani med. 11 ; s. xiii, xiv, No. 8 (Inscribed
   the same as Cusani No. 2)

Erfurt : Amplon. F 236 ; s. xiv, f. 7 (De virtutibus cibariorum.
   Inc. Sicut dixit Gal. Quia corpora hominum. Expl.
   omne nimis ventosus)

Leipzig : Lipsiens. bibl. univ. Repos. med. I 16 ; s. — (Gal.
   liber regiminis sive de cibariis et cibis)

London : Addit. (Br. Mus.) 18, 210 ; s. xiii, xiv, f. 77 (Inscribed
   the same as Amplon. Expl. numdum stringunt
   ventrem)

   Sloan. 1313 ; s. xv, f. 22 (De diff. cib.)

Metz : Mediomatric. 178 ; s. xiv, No. 3 (Inscr. the same as
   London Addit.)

Munich : Monacens. 490 ; a. 1488–1503 (Inscr. the same as
   London Addit.)

Oxford : Coll. Merton. 218 ; s. xiv, f. 206 (De virtutib.
   naturalibus cibarior.)

Paris :   Parisin. 6865 ; s. xiv, f. 194a (Transl. de arab. in lat.
in urbe per magistrum Accursivum Pistoriensem).
Inscr. De virtutibus ciborum (vide Cusani I No. 2)
Nouv. acq. 343 ; s. xiii, f. 74 (Inscr. De cibis. Inc.
Hebet attrahitque succum sibi multum. Fine
mutil.)
Bibl. Univ. 128 ; s. xiv, xv (De cibis)
Rome :   Palat. 1098 ; s. xv, f. 25 (Corresponds with Amplon.)
Vatic. 265 ; s. xii, f. 145 (De. cibis. Inc. Omnia
corpora humana. Expl. as in London,
Addit.)

Latin translations

—   D. I, f. 120 (Guil. de Morbeka interprete)
—   C. I, f. 1082 (Martino Gregorio interprete)
—   Claudii Galeni de alimentorum facultatibus libri III . . .
J. Martinio interprete.   Apud S. Colinæum : Parisiis, 1530.
4°   *540 f. 4 (2)* [B.M.]
—   Claudii Galeni de alimentorum facultatibus libri III.
Ex M. Gregorii interpretatione ; pluribus in locis, hac editione,
emendata. Subjunctus est, alimentorum de quibus agit, index et
monemclator Græcus, Latinus, Gallicus, Belgicus.   Lugduni
Batavorum, 1638.   12°   *349 a. 8* [B.M.]

(39)

περί εὐχυμίας καὶ κακοχυμίας τροφῶν

De probis pravisque alimentorum sucis

Greek and Latin MSS. survive.

Latin MSS.

Bamberg : Bibl. publ. 1691 (L III 37) ; s. xv
Cesena : Malatest. S V 4 ; s. xiv, f. 141 (Inscr. De præser-
vatione a cacochimia)
S XXVI 4 ; s. xiii, f. 90
Dresden : Dresd. Db 92, 93 ; s. xv, f. 312c

Paris : Parisin. 6865 ; s. xiv, f. 186a

Rome : Vatic. 2384* ; s. —, f. 90 (Ex lib. de euchimia et
cacosia)

              2396 ; s. —, f. 243 (Inscr. De rebus boni malive
succi. Inc. Continua serie non paucis
annis. Expl. et longum tempus duravit)

Latin translations

  — D. I, f. 140

  — C. I, f. 1172 (Inscr. Claudii Galeni de Cibis & mali Succi,
Ferdinando Balamio Siculo Interprete. Inc. Annonæ caritas
assidua, quæ non paucos abhinc annos. Expl. quæ cacœthe
appellant, & eius generis acutæ febres, quæ denuo ad tempus
reuertantur)

  — Claudii Galeni Pergameni de euchymia et cacochymia,
seu de bonis malisque succis generandis, J. Guinterio . . .
interprete. Adjectus est Psellii commentarius de victus ratione.
(Per G. Vallam). Parisiis, 1530. 8° *540 b. 12 (4)* [B.M.]

  — Claudii Galeni de bono et malo succo liber unus a S.
Scrofa in Latinum conversus, multisque in locis castigatus
et explicatus. Parisiis, 1546. 8° *540 d. 1 (2)* [B.M.]

  — Another edition. Adscripsimus . . . in margine, scholia ;
brevemq. de cibo et potu, ex Fuchsio assumptam disputationem
. . . adjecimus. MS. notes. Lugduni, 1547. 8° *540 a. 4 (2)*
[B.M.]

(40)

περὶ πτισάνης

De ptisana

Of the MSS. the Greek are known.

Latin translations

  — C. I, f. 1216 (Joanne Polito interprete)

  — M. de Lucio . . . in librum Galeni de ptissana, commentaria . . . cum quæstione de bonitate aquarum earundemque
natura. Venetiis, 1575. 8° *540 b. 14 (3)* [B.M.]

De ptisana—Appendix

— See MERLET (J.) Paraenesis ad medicos antimoniales, ex libro Galeni περὶ πτισάνης. 1655. 4° *1179 h. 13 (1)* [B.M.]

(41)

περὶ τῆς ἐξ ἐνυπνίων διαγνώσεως

De dignotione ex insomniis

The Greek and Latin MSS. are known.

Latin MSS.

Cesena : Malatest. S V 4 ; s. xiv, f. 26

            S XXVI 4 ; s. xviii, f. 13

Chartres : Autricens. 293 (351) ; s. xiv, f. 125

Dresden : Dresd. Db 92, 93 ; s. xv, f. 42c (Inscr. De sompniis)

Erfurt : Amplon. F 236 ; s. xiv (Inscr. De somniis)

Madrid : Matrit. bibl. nac. 1978 (ol. L 60) ; s. xiv, f. 93

Oxford : Oxon. Coll. Omn. Animar. 68 ; s. xiv, f. 190

Paris : Parisin. 6865 ; s. xiv, f. 124b

           7015 ; s. xiv

           7337 ; s. xv (Inscr. De somniis)

Rome : Palat. 1089 ; s. —, f. 114

         1098 ; s. xv, f. 20

         1111 ; s. — (Inscr. De somniis)

      Vatic. 2385 ; s. —, f. 167

Latin translations

— D. I, f. 144

— C. II, f. 1656 (Inscr. Claud. Galeni Dinotione ex Insomniis Libellus, Jano Cornario Medico interprete)

— Claudii Galeni de ea quæ ex insomniis havetur affectionum dignotione, J. Velsio interprete.

— See Hippocrates. [Περὶ Ἐνυπνίων] Hippocratis Col de insomniis liber . . . quinti Hippocratis aphorismi vera lectio, Galeni enarratio &c. 1541. 8° *539 b. 7 (1)* [B.M.]

— Galeni de insomniis liber. Guinterio Andernaco interprete. See Ferrier (A.). A. Ferrerii . . . liber de somniis &c. 1549. 16° *1039 a. 10* [B.M.]

De insomniis—Greek and Latin

— De ea quæ ex insomniis habetur affectionum dignotione See VELSIUS (Justus). Utrum in medico variarum artium et scientiarium cognitio requiratur &c. 1543. 4° *541 c. 24 (2)* [B.M.]

(42)

περὶ διαφορᾶς νοσημάτων
De differentiis morborum

Greek, Arabic, and Hebrew MSS. survive.

Latin translations

— C. II, f. 159 (Nicolao Leoniceno interprete)

— Claudii Galeni . . . de differentiis morborum liber (G. COPO . . . interprete). Edited by J. Struthius. MS. notes. Apud H. Victorem; Cracoviæ, 1537. 8° *7321 aaa 19* [B.M.]
32 leaves without pagination : Sig. A–D.

— Claudii Galeni . . . de morborum et symptomatum differentiis et causis libri sex, G. Copo . . . interprete. Accurata demum cum vetustis codicibus collatione quam plurimis in locis castigati. MS. notes. Lugduni. 1547. 8° *540 a. 3 (1)* [B.M.]

— Commentarii in sex Galeni libros de morbis et symptomatis. F. Valleriola . . . autore. (G. Copo interprete.) [i.e. De morborum differentiis liber, de morborum causis liber, De symptomatum differentiis liber and De symptomatum causis libri tres, with the text in Latin.] (Oratio de re medica . . . F. Valleriola autore.) Venetiis, 1548. 8° *540 d. 32* [B.M.]

— J. F. Rosselli . . . ad sex libros Galeni de differentiis, et causis morborum (N. Leoniceno interprete) et symptomatum

(T. Linacro interprete) commentarii . . . (with the text Latin)
Volumen primum. Hinc subjunctæ sunt ejusdem authoris
(Rosselli) epistolæ &c. 2 parts. Barcinonæ, 1627 fol. *540 h. 18*
[B.M.]

— Claudii Galeni de differentiis morborum liber I. De
causis morborum liber I. (N. Leoniceno interprete.) MS. notes.
Parisiis. 1528. 8° *541 a. 9 (2)* [B.M.]

— Galeni . . . de symptomatum differentiis liber unus.
Ejusdem de symptomatum causis libris tres. T. Lincaro . . .
interprete. Few MS. notes. Londini in ædibus Pynsonianis.
1524. 4° *540 e. 6 (3)* [B.M.]

Without pagination.

— Another edition. Claudii Galeni Pergameni de differentiis
symptomatum. Parisiis, 1528. 8° *541 a. 9 (3)* [B.M.]

De Morbis et Symptomatibus—Appendix

— See Du Bois (J.). Methodus sex librorum Galeni in
differentiis et causis morborum et symptomatum in tabellas sex
. . . conjecta &c. 1539 fol. *540 h. 12* [B.M.]

— See JÆGER (J. G.) Liber Galeni de Symptomatum causis
primus ; in theses contractus &c. 1631. 4° *T. 598 (5)* [B.M.]

— See NUNEZ DE ZAMORA (A.) Repetitiones super caput
primum et tertium libri de differentiis symptomatum Galeni &c.
1621. 4° *540 e. 13 (2)* [B.M.]

— See PONCE DE SANTA CRUZ (A.) A. Ponze Sancta-Crucis
Operum t[omus] III. [A commentary on Galen's works : " De
morborum differentiis, de morborum causis, de symptomatum
differentiis and de symptomatum causis."] 1637 fol. *542 g.
15 (1)* [B.M.]

— See SANTORELLO (A.). J. F. Rosselli censura [of Galen's
six books " de differentiis et causis morborum " &c.] ad censuram
vocata &c. 1628. 4° *1185 k. 1 (2)* [B.M.]

— See SEBISCH (M.) the Younger. Libri sex Galeni de
Morborumdifferentiis, morborumcausis, symptomatum differentiis

et causis. Accesserunt Problemata phlebotomica ex Galeni libro de curandi ratione per sanguinis missionem deprompta, et Dissertatio de Plethora et Cacochymia authore eodem. 1632 &c. 4° *1179 i. 5 (1–8)* [B.M.]

— See WOLFFIUS (Joannes) of Frankfort. Liber Galeni de Symptomatum causis tertius : in these contractus &c. 1632. 4° *T. 598 (7)* [B.M.]

— Methodus sex librorum Galeni in differentiis et causis morborum et symptomatum, in tabellas sex ordine suo conjecta. De signis omnibus medicis, hoc est, salubribus, insalubribus, et neutris, commentarius . . . per J. Sylvium. Parisiis, 1561. 8° *540 c. 13 (1)* [B.M.]

(43)

περὶ τῶν ἐν τοῖς νοσήμασιν αἰτίων

De morborum causis

Greek, Arabic, and Hebrew MSS. are known.

Latin translations

— Usually published together with " De differentiis morborum ", " De symptomatum differentiis ", and " De symptomatum causis libri III ". These six books, as found in the British Museum, have been described together with their catalogue numbers, under section (42) preceding.

— C. II, f. 173 (Nicolao Leoniceno interprete)

(44)

περὶ τῆς τῶν συμπτωμάτων διαφορᾶς

De symptomatum differentiis

Greek, Syriac, Arabic, and Latin MSS. are known.

Latin MSS.

Cambridge : Cantabr. Caius Coll. 948 ; s. —
Oxford : Coll. Merton. 685 ; s. —
Paris : Parisin. 6865 (?) ; s. xiv

Latin translations

— C. II, f. 185 (Thoma Linacro Anglo interprete)
— See remark under *sect.* (*43*) *Latin translations*

(45)

περὶ αἰτίων συμπτωμάτων βιβλία γ′
De symptomatum causis libri III

Greek, Arabic, and Hebrew MSS. are known.

Latin translations

— C. II, f. 197 (Thoma Linacro interprete)
— See remark under *sect.* (*43*) *Latin translations*

(46)

περὶ διαφορᾶς πυρετῶν βιβλία β′
De differentiis febrium libri II

Greek, Arabic, and Latin MSS. are known.

Latin MSS.

Angers : Andecavens. 461 (446) ; s. xvi, f. 34 (Book I,
            annotated by Johanne Riolani)
Basle : Basil. D I 5 ; s. —
Bourges : Biturigens. 299 (247) ; s. xiv, f. 78
Breslau : Vratisl. bibl. univ. IV F 25 ; s. xiii, f. 47*
Cambridge : Cantabr. St. Petri 33 ; s. xiii/xiv, f. 176b
Cesena : Malatest. D XXVI 1 ; s. xiii
                 S V 4 ; xiv, f. 121
                 S XXVII 4 ; s. xiv, no. 10 (Leontii
                       Bononiens. expos.)
Chartres : Autricens. 293 (351) ; s. xiv, f. 86
Cues : Bibl. Nic. Cusani med. 8 ; s. xiii, xiv, No. 7
                        med. 11 ; s. xiii/xiv, No. 7
Erfurt : Amplon. F 249 ; s. xiii, f. 126
              Q 192 ; s. xiv, f. 87

Florence : Laurent. plut. 73, 11* ; s. xiv, f. 54

Madrid : Matrit. bibl. nac. 1198 (ol. L 9) ; s. xiv, f. 151
1978 (ol. L 60) ; s. xiv, f. 83
3308 (ol. L 94) ; s. xv, f. 1

Munich : Monacens. 11 ; s. xiv, f. 36
13026 (Rat. civ. 26) ; s. xiv, f. 87 (sine
auct. nomine)

Naples : Neapol. VIII D 34 ; s. xiv

Oxford : Coll. Balliol. 231 ; s. xiv in. f. 193

Paris : Bibl. de l'Arsenal. 1024 ; s. xiv, f. 165
Parisin. 15455 ; s. xiii, f. 148

Regensburg : Bibl. urb. 47 ; s. xv in.

Rome : Palat. 1092 ; s. —, f. 145
1093 ; s. xiv, f. 138
1094 ; s. xiv, f. 433
1095 ; s. xiv, f. 105
1096 ; s. xiv, f. 116
Urbin. 235 ; s. xiv, f. 151
247 ; s. xiv, f. 193
Vatic. 2375 ; s. xiv, f. 457
2378 ; s. —, f. 229
2381 ; s. —, f. 1
2382 ; s. —, f. 1
2384 ; s. —, f. 68 bis
2386 ; s. —, f. 19
2388 ; s. —, f. 99
4432 ; s. —, f. 81
4451 ; s. xiv, f. 134

Venice : Marcian. App. cl. XIV 6 ; s. xiv, f. 1
26* ; s. xv, f. 66

Volterra : Volaterran. 102 (6365) ; s. xv, f. 90

Latin translations

— D. II, f. 26

— C. II, f. 253 (Inscr. Claud. Galeni De differentiis febrium libri duo ad fidem Codicum Græcorum recogniti, Nicolao. Leoniceno Interprete)

— Galeni de differentiis fœbrium libri duo, interprete L. Laurentiano. Few MS. notes. In officina H. Stephani : Parisiis, 1512. 4° *540 f. 4 (1)* [B.M.]

— Another edition MS. notes. Parisiis, 1519 fol. With Archbishop Cranmer's autograph. *539 h. 5 (2)* [B.M.]

— Thomo de garbo Florentini . . . in libros de Differentiis febrium Galeni Commentu . . . perutile : (with the text in three different Latin translations, one of them that of L. Laurentianus) a proprio exemplari nuper impressum. G.L. Venetiis, 1521, fol. *540 L. 7 (1)* [B.M.]

— Claudii Galeni . . . de differentiis febrium libri duo, L. Laurentiano . . . interprete . . . per S. Thomam recogniti, et ex fide Græci exemplaris pene alii facti. Copious MS. notes. S. Colinæus. Parisiis, 1535 fol. *540 C. 10 (1)* [B.M.]

— Another edition. Few MS. notes. Parisiis, 1539. 8° *540 a. 2 (1)* [B.M.]

— Another edition. MS. notes. Lugduni, 1548. 8° *540 a. 3 (2)* [B.M.]

— Another edition. MS. notes. Lugduni, 1570. 8° *540 a. 3 (3)* [B.M.]

— In Claudii Galeni . . . libros de febribus commentarius, quæ ad febrium cognitionem spectant universa ferme complectens, H. Gibalto, autore. MS. notes. Lugduni, 1562. 8° *540 a. 26* [B.M.]

— Commentaria in librcs Galeni de differentia febrium (with the text). Authore F. Vallesio. Compluti, 1569. 8° *539 C. 24 (2)* [B.M.]

— C. A. Vega . . . commentaria in librum I (–2) Galeni

de differentia febrium (with the text). See VEGA (C. A.) C. A. Vega opera omnia &c. 1626 fol. *542 i. 4* [B.M.]

De Differentiis Febrium—Appendix

— See PAUL of ÆGINA. Pauli Æginetæ . . . de febribus . . . ex Galeni et aliorum commentariis liber unus &c. 1546. 8° *540 C. 18* [B.M.]

— See PLANERO (G.) J. Planerii . . . febrium omnium simplicium divisio . . . ex Galeno . . . excerpta &c. 1574 4° *543 b. 6 (2)* [B.M.]

— Explanationes in Galeni libros de differentiis febrium, item in priorem librum de arte curandi (by V. Trincavellius). See Trincavellius V. V. Trincavelli . . . omnia opera &c. Tom. 1. pt. 1. 1586 fol. *542 i. 2* [B.M.]

(47)

περὶ τῶν ἐν ταῖς νόσοις καιρῶν

De morborum temporibus

The Greek MSS. are known. A single Latin MS. (Parisin. 6861 (?)) has been mentioned.

Latin translations

— C. II, f. 451 (Joanne Guinterio Andernaco interprete)

(48)

περὶ τῶν ὅλου τοῦ νοσήματος καιρῶν

De totius morbi temporibus

Greek and Latin MSS. are known.

Latin MSS.

Cesena : Malatest. S V 4 ; s. xiv, f. 32
                        S XXVI 4 ; s. xiii, f. 15

Chartres : Autricens. 293 (351) ; s. xiv, f. 126 (De temporibus utilibus egenis)

Madrid : Matrit. bibl. nac. 1978 (ol. L 60) ; s. xiv, f. 102
Paris : Parisin. 6865 ; s. xiv, f. 76d
Rome : Vatic. 2376 ; s. —, f. 176

Latin translations

— D. II, f. 37

— C. II, f. 465 (Inscr. Claud. Galeni De totrius morbi
temporibus liber, Joanne Guinterio Andernaco interprete.
Argumenta capitum libri Galeni de Temporibus totius Morbi ;
quæ etian universalia tempora vocat. Reperiuntur autem in
omnibus morbis ; ut particularia tempora (de quibus superiore
libro egit) in periodicis tatum, quales sunt fevres omnes synochis
exceptis. Omnino autem hic libera præcedente separari non debet,
sed pars eius existimari, cum ambos Galenus pro uno libro
scripsisse videatur : proinde communis priori titulus est de
morborum temporibus &c.)

(49)

περὶ τύπων

De typis

The Greek MSS. are known.

Latin translations

— D. II, f. 21 (Nicolao de Regio interprete)

— C. II, f. 475 (Joanne Guinterio Andernaco Medico
interprete)

(50)

πρὸς τοὺς περὶ τύπων γράφαντας, ἢ περὶ περιόδων

Greek MSS. survive at Milan (Ambros. I, 3 sup. ; s. xv, f. 212),
and Paris (Parisin. 2170 ; s. xvi, f. 248)

(51)

περὶ πλήθους

De plenitudine

Greek MSS. are known.

Latin translations

— Claudii Galeni . . . liber de plenitudine ; Polybus de salubri victus ratione privatorum, Guinterio Joanne Andernaco interprete. Apuleius Platonicus de herbarum virtutibus. A. Benivenii libellus de abditis nonnullis ac mirandis morboru. et sanationum causis. 2 parts. Apud Christianum Wechel. [Paris]. 1528 fol. *540 h. 3 (1)* [B.M.]

— Another copy. Few MS. notes. *441 f. 1* [B.M.]

(52)

περὶ τρόμον καὶ παλμοῦ καὶ σπασμοῦ καὶ ῥιγους

De tremore, palpitatione, convulsione et rigore

Greek and Latin MSS. are known.

Latin MSS.

Bourges : Biturigens. 299 (247) ; s. xiv, f. 175 (fine mutil.)
Cambridge : Cantabr. St. Petri 33 ; s. xiii/xiv, f. 169
Cesena : Malatest. S V 4 ; s. xiv, f. 1
                S XXVI 4 ; s. xiii, f. 1
                S XXVII 4 ; s. xiv, No. 7 (Anon. expos.)
Leipzig : Lipsiens. Bibl. Univ. Repos. med. I 4* ; s. — (De
          tremore cordis)
          I 22 ; s. —
Oxford : Coll. Balliol. 231 ; s. xiv, in f. 256b
         Coll. Merton, 230 ; s. xiv, f. 45
Paris : Parisin. 11860 ; s. xiv, f. 238
              15456 ; s. xiii, f. 151
Rome : Palat. 1094 ; s. xiv, f. 451
            1298 ; s. —, f. 219
     Vatic. 2376 ; s. —, f. 193
            2378 ; s. —, f. 208

Latin translations

— D. II, f. 22ᵛ (Petro de Ebano interprete)
— C. II, f. 321 (Jano Cornario Medico Interprete)

(53)

περὶ τοῦ παρ' Ἱπποκράτει κώματος

De comate secundum Hippocratem

A Greek and a Latin MS. are known.   The Latin MS. is
Parisin. 6865 ; s. xiv, f. 198d

Latin translations

— D. II, f. 40 (Nicolao de Regio interprete)
— C. II, f. 315 (Inscr. Claud. Galeni De comate apud Hippocratem Liber, Jano Cornario Medico Physico interprete)

(54)

περὶ μαρασμοῦ

De marcore

Greek, Arabic, and Latin MSS. are known.

Latin MSS.

  Cesena :   Malatest. S V 4 ;   s. xiv, f. 136
                     S XXVI 4 ;   s. xiii, f. 84
  Dresden :   Dresd. Db 92, 93 ;   s. xiv, f. 461d
  Erfurt :   Amplon. F 236 ;   s. xiv, f. 16
  Metz :   Mediomatric. 178 ;   s. xiv, No. 2
  Munich :   Monacens. 490 ;   a. 1488–1503
  Oxford :   Coll. Corp. Christ. 125* ;   s. xiv, xv, xiii, f. 13b
  Paris :   Parisin. 6865 ;   s. xiv, f. 121b
  Rome :   Palat.   1094 ;   s. xiv, f. 632
                 1095 ;   s. xiv, f. 1
          Vatic.   2378 ;   s. —, f. 340
                 2381 ;   s. —, f. 206
                 2384 ;   s. —, f. 64

Latin translations

— D. II, f. 34
— C. II, f. 301 (Inscr. Claudii Galeni De Marasmo, sive
Marcore Liber, Jano Cornario Medico Physico interprete)

(55)

περὶ τῶν παρὰ φύσιν ὄγκων

De tumoribus prætor naturam

Greek, Arabic, and Latin MSS. are known.

Latin MSS.

Cesena : Malatest. S V 4 ; s. xiv, f. 128

              S XXVI 4 ; s. xiii, f. 63

Paris : Parisin. 6865 ; s. xiv, f. 54c

      Nouv. acq. 343 ; s. xiii, f. 50

Rome : Palat. 1098 ; s. xv, f. 43

       Vatic. 2376 ; s. —, f. 206

            2378 ; s. —, f. 225

Latin translations

— D. II, f. 56 (Nicolao de Regio interprete)

— C. II, f. 443 (Horatio Limano interprete)

— See SEBISCH (M.) the Younger. Liber Galeni de tumoribus præter naturam : in theses redactus a M. Sebizio &c. Argentorat : 1633. 4° *1179 i. 5 (10)* [B.M.]

— C. Galeni . . . De tumoribus præternaturam liber. Guinterio Joanne Andernaco interprete. Pariis, 1529. 8° *540 b. 12 (3)* [B.M.]

(56)

περὶ ἀνωμάλου δυσκρασίας

De inæquali intemperie

Greek, Arabic, Hebrew, and Latin MSS. are known.

Latin MSS.

Angers : Andecavens. 461 (446) ; s. xvi, f. 7

Cesena : Malatest. S V 4 ; s. xiv, f. 135

             S XXVI 4 ; s. xiii, f. 80

Erfurt : Amplon. F 278 ; s. xiv in f. 171

Madrid : Matrit. bibl. nac. 1978 (ol. L 60) ; s. xiv, f. 91

                   3308 (ol. L 94) ; s. xv, f. 158

Metz : Mediomatric. 178 ; s. xiv, No 4
Munich : Monacens. 490 ; a 1488–1503
Oxford : Coll. Merton, 685
Paris : Parisin. 6765 (?)

Latin translations
— D. I, f. 42
— C. II, f. 293 (Thoma Linacro Anglo interprete)

Inc. Argumenta capitum libri Galeni de inæquali intemperie, secundum Joannem Agricolam, qui commentarios scripsit, & in duodecim capita hunc librum diuidit; aliqui novem tantum faciunt, quorum distinctionem ciphra denotat in contextu.

— Liber aureus de inæquali intemperie, Latinitate donatus a T. Linacro. Cui . . . familiares adjecit commentraios J. Agricola Ammonius. Accedunt huc alia plura &c. (Concordantiæ in autores præcipuos simplicium medicamentorum. In quibus primo statim aspectu deprehenditur, num aliquo, et in quo loco simplex quodque descripserint Dioscorides, Galenus et Serapio. Epicedion I. Marschalchi in Bappenheim . . . absolbit et elaboravit G. Leonbergerus. Ad scholiomastiga apologia ; ad J. Gengerum epistole de variis rebus medicis. (By J. Agricola Ammonius.) Hippocratis Jusjurandum cum libello de lege. Few MS. notes. Basileæ, 1539. 8° *540 b. 2* [B.M.]

— In Claudii Galeni . . . librum de inæquali intemperie commentarii A. Busennii (with the text). Antverpiæ, 1553. 8° *774 b. 10 (2)* [B.M.]

De inæquali intemperie—Appendix

— See CALANIUS (P.) P. Calani Paraphrasis in Galenum de inæquali intemperie. 1538. 8° *540 d. 16* [B.M.]

This work inscribed *De malitia complexionis diversæ*, was published in the Giunta edition of Galen (1528, II, f. 42).

The *Latin MSS.* are :—

Basle : Basil. D I 5 ; s. —
Bourges : Biturigens. 299 (247) ; s. xiv, f. 144

Breslau : Vratisl. bibl. univ. IV F 25 ; s. xiii, f. 125–7
                 IV F 26 ; s. —, 86–8

Brügge : Bibl. publ. 466 ; s. xiii

Cambrai : nr. 907 (806) ; s. xiv, f. 164

Cambridge : Cantabr. St. Petri 33 ; s. xiii/xix, f. 23b

Cesena : Malatest. D XXV 1 ; s. xiii, f. 56
              D XXV 2 ; s. xiii
              S V 4 ; s. xiv, f. 117

Chartres : Autricens. 284 (340) ; s. xiii, f. 62
               293 (351) ; s. xiv, f. 56

Cues : Bibl. Nic. Cusani med. 8 ; s. xiii, xiv, No. 8
                     11 ; s. xiii/xiv, No. 5

Eton : Bibl. Coll. 132 ; s. xiii, No. 13

Erfurt : Amplon. F 249 ; s. xiii, f. 234
           Q 178* ; s. xiii

London : Addit. (Br. Mus.) 22, 669 ; s. xiv, f. 45
        Harleian. 3748 ; s. xv, f. 208
               5425 ; s. xiii, f. 53

Montpellier : Montepess. (École de Méd.) 18 ; s. xiii

Munich : Monacens. 5 ; s. xiv, f. 143
               11 ; s. xiv, f. 94
              3512 (Aug. civ.) 12 ; a. 1300, f. 337

Naples : Neapol. VIII D 30 ; s. xiv
          VIII D 34 ; s. xiv

Oxford : Coll. Balliol. 231 ; s. xiv in f. 280b
        Coll. Merton. 218 ; s. xiv, f. 25
                219 ; s. xiv in f. 36b (early 14th cent.)

Paris : Bibl. de l'Arsenal 1080* ; s. xiv, f. 24 (abbreviat. a
    Joh. de St. Amando)

Parisin.   6765 (?)
                    6865 ; s. xiv, f. 152c
                    7015 ; s. xiv
                  11860 ; s. xiv, f. 82
                  14389 ; s. xiv
                  15455 ; s. xiii, f. 94
nouv. acq.   343 ; s. xiii, f. 37
                    1482 ; s. —, f. 76
Rome : Palat. 1092 ; s. —, f. 19
                  1093 ; s. —, f. 125
                  1094 ; s. xiv, f. 85
                  1095 ; s. xiv, f. 51
                  1096 ; s. xiv, f. 126
        Urbin.   209 (ol. 285)* ; s. xiv–xv, f. 119
                  247 ; s. xiv, f. 85
        Vatic. 2375 ; s. xiv, f. 24
                  2378 ; s. —, f. 60
                  2381 ; s. —, f. 196
                  2386 ; s. —, f. 48 (?)
                  2416 ; s. —, f. 58
Venice : Marcian. App. cl. XIV 5 ; s. xiv, f. 49
                                26* ; s. xv, f. 65
Volterra : Volterran. 103 (6365) ; s. xv, f. 87

(57)

περὶ δυσπνοίας βιβλία γ'

De difficultate respirationis libri III

Greek and Latin MSS. are known.

Latin MSS.

Cesena : Malatest. S V 4 ; s. xiv, f. 150
                    S XXVI 4 ; s. xiii, f. 108
Dresden : Dresd. Db 92, 93 ; s. xv, f. 451b
Paris : Parisin. 6865 ; s. xiv, f. 200c

Latin translations
— D. II, f. 41 (Nicolao de Regio interprete)
— C. II, f. 341 (Jano Cornario Medico interprete)
— De difficultate respirationis. [Translated by J. Cornarius.]
See Marcellus, Empiricus. Marcelli de medicamentis empiricis
liber &c. 1531 fol. *539 k. 16 (1–5)* [B.M.]

(58)

περὶ τῶν πεπονθότων τόπων βιβλία ζ'

De locis affectis libri VI

Greek, Arabic (Syriac ?), and Latin MSS. are known.

Latin MSS.

Boulogne-sur-Mer : Bononiens. 197 ; s. xiii, No. 1 (Expl. et
                           passionem ostendunt)
Breslau : Vratisl. bibl. univ. IV F 25 ; s. xiii, f. 105–25
                            IV F 26 ; s. —, f. 17–46
Cambridge : Cantabr. Caius Coll. 98 ; s. xv, f. 113 (Expl. in
                            essentia cerebri)
             St. Petri 33 ; s. xiii/xiv, f. 94b
Cesena : Malatest. D XXV 1 ; s. xiii, f. 113
             S V 4 ; s. xiv, f. 77
Erfurt : Amplon. F 249 ; s. xiii, f. 25
             F 278 ; s. xiv, in f. 84
Eton : Bibl. Coll. 132 ; s. xiii, No. 4
Laon : Laudemens. 421 ; s. xiii, No. 1 (Inscr. " Gal Anatomia ")
Leipzig : Lipsiens. bibl. univ. Repos. med. I 4 ; s. —
                               II 49 ; s. —(Lectt.
                               in Gal. libb.)
London : Harleian (Br. Mus.) 3748 ; s. xv, f. 135 (Expl. in
                            suo loco dicemus)
                         5425 ; s. xiii, f. 56 (Sine inscr.
                            . . . Expl. quare residuum
                            . . . ponosticorum)
         Regius 12 C XV ; s. xiii, f. 86

Madrid : Matrit. bibl. nac. 1198 (ol. L 9) ; s. xiv, f. 16

Montecassino : Casinens. 70 ; s. xiv, p. 163

Montpellier : Montepess (École de méd.) 18 ; s. xiii

Munich : Monacens.   5 ; s. xiv, f. 61

                35 ; s. xiii, xiv, f. 61 (Libri III–VI)

                3520 (Aug. civ. 20) ; s. xiv, f. 57 (Inc.
                     Quoniam diversitas membrorum
                     corporis)

                13026 (Rat. civ. 26) ; s. xiv, f. 66

Oxford : Coll. Balliol. 231 ; s. xiv in. f. 76 (Expl. similar to
                            Harleian 3748)

        Coll. Merton. 218 ; s. xiv, f. 173 (Expl. vel passionem
                            ostendunt, vide Bononiens
                            197)

        Coll. Merton. 230 ; s. xiv, f. 99 (Inc. similar to Monac.
                            3520. Expl. similar to
                            Cantabr. Caius Coll. 98)

        Coll. Merton. 685 ; s. —

Paris : Bibl. de l'Arsenal 1080 ; s. —, f. 6

      Parisin.   6865A ; s. xiv

               6865B ; s. xiv

               9331 ; s. xv

               11860 ; s. xiv, f. 125

               14389 ; s. xiv, f. 105

               15455 ; s. xiii, f. 23

               Nouv. acq. 1482 ; s. —, f. 2

Perugia : Perusian. 44 (A 44) ; s. xv, f. 22–8 (Inc. " Intentio
       Galeni ". Expl. point quandum narrationem)

Regensburg : Bibl. urb. 46 ; s. —, (Libri II)

                    69 ; s. —

Rome : Palat.   1093 ; s. xiv, f. 1

               1094 ; s. xiv, f. 288

               1184 ; s. —, f. 112

Urbin.   235 ;   s. xiv, f. 103
247 ;   s. xiv, f. 254

Vatic.   2375 ;   s. xiv, f. 161
2378 ;   s. —, f. 173
2379 ;   s. —, f. 64
2381 ;   s. —, f. 12
2383 ;   s. —, f. 78
2385 ;   s. —, f. 1
2389 ;   s. —, f. 21
4467 ;   s. —, f. 33

Vendôme : Vindocin. 234 ; s. xiv, f. 43 (Expl. nec. tumorem nec . . .)

Venice : Marcian. cl. XIV, 6 ; s. xiv, f. 23
7 ; s. xiv, f. 41 (L I cap. i)

Volterra : Volaterran. 103 (6365) ; s. xv, f. 27

Wolfenbüttel : Guerferbyt. 1615 (I. 8. Aug.) ; s. xiv, f. 244–67

There are no Syriac or Hebrew MSS. extant.

Latin translations

— D. II, f. 58
— C. II, f. 829 (Gulielmo Copo Basiliensi Interprete)
— Giunta ed. (1525), II, f. 58
— Galeni de affectorum locorum notitia libri VI. G. Copo
. . . interprete. MS. notes.

J. Hertzog ? Venice, 1510 ? fol. *543 g. 21 (1)* [B.M.]

— Another edition. Copious MS. notes.

H. Estienne. Paris, 1513. 5° *540 e. 5 (2)* [B.M.]

Imperfect : wanting title page ; leaf A ii is mutilated.

— Another edition. Ex secunda recognitione. Few MS. notes. In officina Simonis Colinæi. Parisiis, 1520 fol. *7320 h. 7* [B.M.]

— Another edition. Ex tertia recognitione. MS. notes. Parisiis, 1539. 8° *540 a. 2 (2)* [B.M.]

— Another edition. Cum . . . commentariis J. F. Duratii. Venetiis, 1557. 8° *774 b. 11* [B.M.]

Contains only books 1–3.

— Another copy. *540 b. 5 (1)* [B.M.]

— Claudii Galeni de locorum affectorum notitiæ . . . recogniti brevique . . . expositione marginali . . . illustrati. Lugduni, 1562. 8° *774 a. 10 (3)* [B.M.]

De locis affectis—Appendix

— See GERCIA CARRERO (P.). Disputationes medicæ super libros Galeni de locis affectis &c. 1605 fol. *776 m. 7* [B.M.]

— De locis affectis. See Strobelberger (J. S.) Prælectionem Monspeliensium a J. S. Strobelbergero in Monte Palio . . . habitarum . . . recapitulatio continens . . . Summariam libri primi Galeni de affectorum locorum notitia explanationem. 1625 ? 12° *731 a. 3 (2)* [B.M.]

— See WOLFIUS (Joannes) Professor at Helmstadt. Exercitationes in Claudii Galeni de locis affectis libros VI &c. 1620. 4° *1179 b. 3 (1–12)* [B.M.]

(59)

περὶ σφυγμῶν τοῖς εἰσαγομένοις

De pulsibus ad Tirones

Greek and Latin MSS. are known.

Latin MSS.

Bourges : Biturigens. 299 (247) ; s. xiv, f. 128

Breslau : Vratislav. IV F 25 ; s. xiii, f. 164–6

Cambridge : Cantabr. St. Petri 33 ; s. xiii/xiv, f. 173

Cesena : Malatest. S V 4 ; s. xiv, f. 59

Dresden : Dresd. Db 92, 93 ; s. xv, f. 30a (a Burgondione jud. Pis. transl.)

Erfurt : Amplon. F 249 ; s. xiii, f. 284

Escurial : Scorial. L. III, 18 ; s. xiii, f. 70

Milan : Ambros. G 108 Inf. ; s. x, f. 92 (Inscr. Peri sfigmon
    Galieni isagogen ad Teuthram)

Montecassino : Casinens. 70 ; s. xiv, p. 154

Moulins : nr. 30 ; s. xiv, f. 86

Munich : Monac. 3512 (Aug. civ. 12) ; a. 1300, f. 334

Oxford : Coll. Balliol. 231 ; s. xiv, in f. 202b (Inscr. De
    differenciis pulsuum)

Paris : Parisin. 7015 ; s. xiv
                11860 ; s. xiv, f. 228
                14389 ; s. xiv, f. 144
                15455 ; s. xiii, f. 158

Rome : Palat. 1094 ; s. xiv, f. 490
              1099 ; s. xv, f. 61
       Urbin. 247 ; s. xiv, f. 318
       Vatic. 2375 ; s. xiv, f. 247
              2376 ; s. —, f. 100
              2378 ; s. —, f. 95
              2383 ; s. —, f. 120
              2384 ; s. —, f. 53

Venice : Marcian. cl. XIV 6 ; s. xiv, f. 56 (c. Comm.)

Latin translations

— D. I, f. 89

— C. II, f. 971 (Hermanno Cruserio Campensi interprete,
Inc. Quæ interest tyronum, charissime Teuthra)

— Claudii   Galeni . . . introductio   in   pulsus . . . M.
Gregorio interprete. See supra. Two or more works. Latin.
Claudii Galeni . . . Introductio &c. 1541. 8° *540 a. 6 (1)*
[B.M.]

— 1550. 8° *540 a. 6 (2)* [B.M.]

— Claudii Galeni de pulsibus ad Tyrones liber . . . in
Latinum sermonem conversus, per F. Menam . . . cum ejusdem
commentariis . . . adjectis passim plurimorum locorum in

libros Galeni de pulsibus castigationibus.　Few MS. notes.
Compluti.　1553.　4°　*540 e. 11 (4)* [B.M.]

This work of Galen was rendered into Arabic by Joannitius
(see ch. 2 of this work), and later translated into Latin by Marcus
of Toledo.　The Latin MSS. are inscribed *De tactu pulsus*.

Inc. Narrabo tibi, karissimi Tutire.

Latin MSS.

Basle : Basil. D III 8 ;　s. —

Bourges : Biturigens. 299 (247) ;　s. xiv, f. 132

Breslau : Vratisl. bibl. univ. IV F 25 ;　s. xiii, f. 162–4 (De
utilitate [tactus] pulsus)

Cambridge : Cantabr. St. Petri 33 ;　s. xiii/xiv, f. 184

Chartres : Autricens. 284 (340) ;　s. xiii, f. 129

Dresden : Dresd. Db. 92, 93 ;　s. xv, f. 34c (Commences " Pro-
hemium Marci Toletani in librum Galieni de
tactu pulsus, quem transtulit de arabico in
latinum et hunc antea transtulerat Johannicius
filius Ysaac de greco in arabicum ").

Erfurt : Amplon. F 249 ;　s. xiii, f. 287
F 276 ;　s. xiv, f. 67

Eton : Bibl. Coll. 132 ;　s. xiii, No. 7

Montpellier : Montepass. (École de méd.) 18 ;　s. xiii

Moulins : nr. 30 ;　s. xiv, f. 82

Oxford : Coll. Balliol. 231 ;　s. xiv, in. f. 45

Paris : Parisin.　6865 ;　s. xiv, f. 207 (Particula 16 libri Mega
pulsus)
11860 ;　s. xiv, f. 222
15455 ;　s. xiii, f. 165

Rome : Palat. 1094 ;　s. xiv, f. 196

(60)

περὶ διαφορᾶς σφυγμῶν λόγοι δ'

De pulsuum differentiis libri IV

Greek, Arabic, and Latin MSS. are known.

Latin MSS.

Breslau : Vratisl. Bibl. Univ. IV F 26 ; s. —, f. 83–6

Cesena : Malatest. D XXIII 1 ; s. xiii

D XXV 2 ; s. xiii

S V 4 ; s. xiv, f. 70

Cues : Bibl. Nic. Cusani med. 11 ; s. xiii, xiv, No. 10

Madrid : Matrit. bibl. nac. 1198 (ol. L 9)* ; s. xiv, f. 165

(Libri 1 pars extr.)

Munich : Monac. 3856 (Aug. eccl. 156) ; s. xiii, f. 128

Paris : Parisin. 6865 ; s. xiv, f. 124c (Lib. I, II a Burgundione

transl.)

7015 ; s. xiv

Rome : Palat. 1099 ; s. xv, f. 37

Vatic. 2375 ; s. xiv

2376 ; s. —, f. 94

2378 ; s. —, f. 91

2383 ; s. —, f. 135

2384 ; s. —, f. 30

2386 ; s. —, f. 1

Vendôme : Vindocin. 240 ; s. xvi, f. 40 (libri II–IV)

Venice : Marcian. cl. XIV 6* ; s. xiv, 66

Latin translations

— D. I, f. 89

— C. II, f. 983 (Hermanno Cruserio Campensi interprete)

(61)

περὶ διαγνώσεως σφυγμῶν λόγοι δ'

De dignoscendis pulsibus libri IV

Greek, Arabic, and Latin MSS. are known.

Latin MSS.

Cesena : Malatest. S V 4 ; s. xiv, f. 75

Rome : Palat. 1099 ; s. xv, f. 61

Vendôme : Vindocin. 240 ; s. xvi, f. 1

Latin translations

— C. II, f. 1065 (Hermanno Cruserio Campensi interprete)

(62)

περὶ τῶν ἐν τοῖς σφυγμοῖς σιτίων λόγοι δ΄

De causis pulsuum libri IV

Greek, Arabic, and Latin MSS. are known.

Latin MSS.

Bourges : Biturigens. 299 (247) ; s. xiv, f. 117

Breslau : Vratisl. bibl. univ. IV F 25 ; s. xiii, f. 157–62 [161a]
      (De causis principalibus alterantibus pulsuum
      III, IV)

Cesena : Malatest. D XXIII, 1 ; s. xiii (De causis pulsuum
              libri IV)

            D XXV, 2 ; s. xiii (Inscr. similar to
              D XXIII, 1)

            S V 4 ; s. xiv, f. 62 (De causis pulsuum)

Munich : Monac. 5 ; s. xiv, f. 243

Oxford : Coll. Balliol 231 ; s. xiv in f. 206b (Inc. " Has
      quidem quæ a primis " [=Inc. lib. III].   Expl.
      spiritus in arteriis proficitur)

Paris : Parisin.   6865 ; s. xiv, f. 130b (Liber III de causis
              pulsus)

           11860 ; s. xiv, f. 291

           15455 ; s. xiii, f. 173 (Liber III, IV)

Rome : Palat.   1099 ; s. xv, f. 46 (Liber III, IV)

      Urbin.   247 ; s. xiv, f. 244

      Vatic.   2375 ; s. xiv, f. 259 (De causis pulsuum liber
              III, IV)

2376 ; s. —, f. 104 (Liber III, IV)
2378 ; s. —, f. 97
2383 ; s. —, f. 124
2384 ; s. —, f. 35
2386 ; s. —, f. 8 (Liber III Megapulsi)

Latin translations

— D. I, f. 91

— C. II, f. 1123 (Hermanno Cruserio Campensi interprete)

— J. A. Ungebaner . . . dissertatio . . . de Pulsu inæquali ad mentum Galeni de Causis Pulsuum Liber II.

See SCHLEGEL (J. C. T.) Thesaurus Semiotices pathologicæ &c. Vol. I. 1787 &c. 8° *773 e. 21* [B.M.]

(63)

περὶ προγνώσεως σφυγμῶν λόγοι δ'

De præsagitione ex pulsibus libri IV

Greek, Arabic, and Latin MSS. are known.

Latin MSS.

Parisin. 6865 ; s. xiv, f. 207a (Particula 16. Megapulsus (=Liber IV). Inc. Osta particula 4a particularum. Expl. omnium sufficientum in libris criseos)

Latin translations

— C. II, f. 1183 (Hermano Cruserio Campensi interprete)

(64)

σύνοψις περὶ σφυγμῶν ἰδίας πραγματείας

Synopsis librorum suorum sedicem de pulsibus

Greek and Latin MSS. are known. A Latin MS. is at Cheltenham (Phillipps, 24, 386 ; s. xv, f. 1)

(65)

περὶ κρίσεων βιβλία γ'

De crisibus libri III

Greek, Arabic, Hebrew, and Latin MSS. are known.

Latin MSS.

Basle : Basil. D III 6 ; s. —

                D III 8 ; s. —

Breslau : Vratisl. bibl. univ. IV F 25 ; s. xiii, f. 186–99

Cambrai : Camaracens. 907 (806) ; s. xiv, f. 113

Cambridge : Cantabr. St. Petri 33 ; s. xiii/xiv, f. 41

Cesena : Malatest. D XXV, 1 ; s. xiii, f. 89 (Libri VI)

Chartres : Autricens. 284 (340) ; s. xiii, f. 228

                    293 (351) ; s. xiv, f. 17

Cues : Bibl. Nic. Cusani med. 1 ; s. xiii, No. 1

                      8 ; s. xiii, xiv, No. 2

Erfurt : Amplonian. F 249 ; s. xiii, f. 138

                F 291 ; s. xiii, ex. f. 46

                Q 178* ; s. xiii

                Q 198 ; s. xiv, in. f. 25

Eton : Bibl. Coll. 132 ; s. xiii, No. 2

Florence : Laurent. plut. 73, 11 ; s. xiv, f. 78

          Laurent. Leopold. (Gaddian.) 58 ; s. xiv, f. 68

Leipzig : Lipsiens. bibl. univ. Repos. med. I 21 ; s. —

                           I 29 ; s. —

London : Harleian (Br. Mus.) 3748 ; s. xv, f. 1

Madrid : Matritens. bibl. nac. 1198 (ol. L 9) ; s. xiv, f. 56

                    1978 (ol. L 60) ; s. xiv, f. 103

Marburg : Bibl. univ. B 2 ; s. xiii, f. 9

Metz : Mediomatric. 178 ; s. xiv, No. 6

Montecassino : Casinens. 70 ; s. xiv, p. 90

Montpellier : Montepess. (École de méd.) 18 ; s. xiii

Munich : Monacens.   5 ; s. xiv, f. 145

                    35 ; s. xiii, xiv, f. 82

              13027 (Rat. civ. 27) ; s. xii/xiv, f. 40

                        (Libri IV)

13054 (Rat. civ. 54) ; s. xiv, f. 31 (Libri
II. c. Comm.) et f. 164 (Nic.
Bononiensis expositio super
libr. II. De crisi)

Naples : Neapolit. VIII D 30 ; s. xiv

Oxford : Coll. Omnium Animarum 68 ; s. xiv, xv, f. 192
Coll. Balliol. 231 ; s. xiv, f. 154b
Bodlei. Canonician. misc. 307 ; s. xiv, ex. f. 121
(Expl. in summo urine aut penduos)
Coll. Merton. 218 ; s. xiv, f. 129
219 ; s. xiv, in. f. 115
685 ; s. —

Padua : Bibl. S. Joannis in Viridario, ad læv. plut. XVIII
(Whereabouts not known)

Paris : Bibl. de l'Arsenal 1080 ; s. xiv, f. 11
Parisin. 6865A ; s. xiv
9331 ; s. xv
11860 ; s. xiv, f. 39
14389 ; s. xiv, f. 177
15455 ; s. xiii, f. 96
nouv. acq. 1482 ; s.—, f. 87

Perugia : Perusin. 44 (A 44) ; s. xv, f. 31–5

Reims : nr. 1014 ; s. xiv, f. 1 (Ambrosii de Berssangiis
expositio super. libr. I et II. Inc. Ego non intendo.
Expl. sufficienter determinat) et f. 65 (Expos.
libri III, edita a mag. Petro de Alvernia. Inc.
Intentio vero. Expl. nihil est possibile videri)

Rome : Palat. 1092 ; s. —, f. 100
1093 ; s. xiv, f. 49
1094 ; s. xiv, f. 356
1095 ; s. xiv, f. 132
1096 ; s. xiv, f. 81^v

Urbin.   247 ; s. xiv, f. 282

Vatic.   2375 ; s. xiv, f. 114

2378 ; s. —, f. 77

2379 ; s. —, f. 98

2381 ; s. —, f. 48

2385 ; s. —, f. 35

2386 ; s. —, f. 97

4451 ; s. xiv, f. 115 (Inc. mutil. : ventris augmentum, hinc crisis erit)

Subiaco : nr. 49 ; s. xiii, f. 39 (anepigr.)

Vendôme : Vindocinens 234 ; s. xiv, f. 21

Volterra : Volaterran. 103 (6365) ; s. xv, f. 1

Wolfenbüttel : Guerferbyt. 2189 (16, 3 Aug.)* ; a. 1440–4. f. 330 (Dictum Gal. De crisi)

Latin translations

— D. I, f. 239

— C. II, f. 1257 (Nicolao Leoniceno interprete)

— Claudii Galeni de crisibus libri tres, Nicolas Leoniceno interprete, nunc ab omnibus . . . mendis repurgati, cum . . . indice in hac ultima impressione adjecto. pp. 192.   Apud G. Rouillium. Lugduni, 1558.   8°   *540 a. 35 (2)* [B.M.]

— Galeni libri de Crisibus, interprete Hieronymo Boniperto . . . Ejus dem Hieronymi quæstio . . . in qua queritur, an expediat humores non concoctos neque duriosos, sed multitudine ac malu etiam qualitate peccateis (*sic*) inter morborum initia cum purgante medicamento minorare, necue &c. 2 pt. Venetiis. 1547.   4°   *C. 66 e. 13* [B.M.]

De Crisibus—Appendix

— See SALVIANI (I.) De crisibus ad Galeni censuram liber &c. 1558.   8°   *540 d. 6 (2)* [B.M.]

(66)

περὶ κρισίμων ἡμερῶν βιβλία γ′

De diebus decretoris libri III

Greek, Arabic, Hebrew, and Latin MSS. are known.

Latin MSS.

Basle : Basil. D. III 8 ; s. —

Bourges : Biturigens. 299 (247) ; s. xiv, f. 22

Breslau : Vratislav. bibl. univ. IV E 25 ; s. xiii, f. 81–91

Cambrai : Camaracens. 907 (806) ; s. xiv, f. 142

Cambridge : Cantabr. St. Petri 33 ; s. xiii/xiv, f. 59

Cesena : Malatest. D XXV, 1 ; s. xiii, f. 50
　　　　　　　　　　S XXVIII, 4 ; s. xiv, No. 8 (Anon. Comm.)

Chartres : Autricens. 284 (340) ; s. xiii, f. 214
　　　　　　　　　　293 (351) ; s. xiv, f. 94

Cheltenham : Phillipps. 6915 ; s. xv (? sold)

Erfurt : Amplonian. F 294 ; s. xiii, f. 165
　　　　　　　　　F 291 ; s. xiii, f. 58
　　　　　　　　　Q 198 ; s. xiv, in. f. 52

Eton : Bibl. Coll. 132 ; s. xiii, No. 1

Florence : Laurent.-Leopold. (Caddian.) 58 ; s. xiv, f. 97

London : Harleian (Br. Mus.) ; s. xv, f. 25

Madrid : Matritens. bibl. nac. 1198 (ol. L 9) ; s. xiv, f. 42
　　　　　　　　　　1978 (ol. L 60) ; s. xiv, f. 108

Marburg : Bibl. univ. B 2 ; s. xiii, f. 32

Montecassino : Casinens. 70 ; s. xiv, p. 51

Montpellier : Montepess. (École de méd.) 18 ; s. xiii

Munich : Monac.　　5 ; s. xiv, f. 168
　　　　　　　13027 (Rat. civ. 27) ; s. xii/xiv, f. 53
　　　　　　　13054 (Rat. civ. 54) ; s. xiv, f. 143 [Nic.
　　　　　　　　　　Bononiensis sup. libr. de criticis]

Naples :   Neapolit. VIII D 30 ;   s. xiv

Oxford :   Balliol. Coll. 231 ;   s. xiv, in. f. 176b
             Canonician. misc. 307 ;   s. xiv, ex. f. 117
             Merton. Coll. 218 ;   s. xiv, f. 154
                             219 ;   s. xiv, in. f. 141

Paris :   Parisin.   7015 ;   s. — (Comm. Nic. de Anglia)
                      9331 ;   s. xv
                      11860 ;   s. xiv, f. 52
                      14389 ;   s. xiv, f. 156
                      15455 ;   s. xiii, f. 130
                      Nouv. acq. 1482 ;   s. —, f. 114

Perugia :   Perusin. 44 (A 44) ;   s. xv, f. 28–31

Rome :   Angelic.   242 (C 4, 10) ;   s. xiv, f. 50 (liber III)
          Palat.   1092 ;   s. —, f. 125
                   1094 ;   s. xiv, f. 331
                   1095 ;   s. xv, f. 115
                   1096 ;   s. xiv, f. 52
          Urbin.   247 ;   s. xiv, f. 174
          Vatic.   2375 ;   s. xiv, f. 135
                   2378 ;   s. —, f. 109
                   2379 ;   s. —, f. 122
                   2381 ;   s. —, f. 74
                   2385 ;   s. —, f. 58
                   2386 ;   s. —, f. 81
                   4451 ;   s. xiv, f. 103 (Libri I et II)

Salamanca :   Bibl. univ. 2–4–6 ;   s. xvii, f. 1 (Ald. Garzeran
             interpr.)

Volterra :   Volaterran. 103 (6365) ;   s. xv, f. 136 (fine mutil.)

Latin translations

— D. I, f. 258
— C. II, f. 1323 (Joanne Guinterio Andernaco interprete)
— Claudii Galeni de diebus decretoriis libri tres, J. Guinterio

. . . interprete. Nuperrime ad exampla Venetum recogniti &c. Lugduni, 1553. 8° *540 a. 7 (2)* [B.M.]

— Claudii Galeni . . . de diebus decretoriis libri III . . . Latini facti et commentariis illustrati . . . J. Lalamantio . . . auctore. Lugduni, 1560, fol. *540 g. 22* [B.M.]

— H. Obicii . . . Commentarius in Claudii Galeni librum tertium de diebus decretoriis (with the text). See Obicius, H. H. Obicii . . . de multiplici in medicina abusu tractatus &c. Part 4. 1618. 4° *542 e. 1* [B.M.]

— Flagellum medicorum astronomiæ imperitorum sive dies juditii, de diebus decretoriis opus tertium . . . Per Messire J. B. Damascene. Parisiis, 1663. 4° *540 e. 13 (3)* [B.M.] Several leaves have been mutilated in binding.

De diebus decretoriis—Appendix

— Commentarius in Claudii Galeni de diebus decretoriis librum tertium. See MAGINI (J. A.). J. A. Magini . . . de Astrologica Ratione ac usu dierum criticorum . . . opus &c. 1607. 4° *718 e. 16* [B.M.]

— 1608. 4° *718 h. 6* [B.M.]

— See PLANERO (G.) J. Planerii . . . I. Dubitationum et solutionum in III. Galeni de diebus criticis liber unus . . . II. In eundem tertium Galeni de diebus criticis scholia &c. 1594. 4° *543 b. 6 (3)* [B.M.]

(67)

θεραπευτικῆς μεθόδου βιβλία ιδ΄

Methodi medendi libri XIV

Greek, Arabic, and Latin MSS. are known.

Latin MSS.

    Angers : Andecavens. 461 (446)* ; s. xvi, f. 81. (J. Riolani annott.)

    Basle : Basil. D I 5 ; s. — (L. VII–XIV)

            D III 8 ; s. — (Megategni)

Boulogne-sur-Mer : nr. 197 ; s. xiii, No. 3 (Megat.)

Breslau : Vratisl. bibl. univ. IV F 25 ; s. xiii, f. 168–86 (Libri
                         VIII)
                         IV F 26 ; s. —, f. 88^v–98^v
                         (L. I–IV)

Cambrai : Camaracens. 907 (806) ; s. xiv, f. 1 (Megat.)

Cambridge : Cantabr. Caius Coll. 98 ; s. xv, f. 7 (Megat.)
                         946, 947, 955 (Megat.)
        St. Johann D 3 ; s. xiii, f. 32 (Megat.)
        St. Petri 33 ; s. xiii/xiv, f. 1 (Megat.) et f. 241b
        (De Ingenio Saint. Inc. Quare tantum distulit)

Cesena : Malatest. D XXIII 1 ; s. xiii (L. I–VI [inscr. De
      diagnosi seu de cognitione morborum] et I
      VII–XIV)
      Malatest. D XXV 2 ; s. xiii
                S   V 4 ; s. xiv, f. 159 (L. VII–XIV)
                et f. 219

Chartres : Autricens. 284 (340) ; s. xiii, f. 80 et f. 164 (Megat.)
               293 (351) ; s. xiv, f. 1 (Megat.) et f. 58

Cues : Bibl. Nic. Cusani med. 8 ; s. xiii, xiv, No. 4
                    11 ; s. xiii, xiv, No. 2

Dresden : Dresd. Db 92, 93 ; s. xv, f. 467a (Megat.) et f. 565c
        (Cura egritudinum)

Erfurt : Amplon. F 249 ; s. xiii, f. 1 (Megat. seu de ing.
        sanitat.)
        F 278 ; s. xiv in. f. 118 (L. VII–XIV)
        Q 219* ; a. 1335, f. 197–200

Eton : Bibl. Coll. 132 ; s. xiii, No. 5 (Megat.) et No. 6 (De
      ingen. sanit.)

Florence : Laurent.-Leopold (Gaddian) 58 ; s. xiv, f. 1

Leipzig : Lipsiens. bibl. univ. Repos. med. I 29 ; s. — (Megat.)

London : Addit. (Br. Mus.) 22, 669 ; s. xiv, f. 1 (L. X–XIV)
        Harleian. 3748 ; s. xv, f. 42
        Regius 12 C XV ; s. xiii, f. 118

Madrid : Matrit. bibl. nac. 1198 (ol. L 9) ; s. xiv, f. 99 (L.
II–XIV ordine librorum pertur-
bato)
1978 (ol. L 60) ; s. xiv, f. 2
(L. VII–XIV)

Montecassino : Casinens. 70 ; s. xiv, p. 291 (L. VII–XIV)

Montpellier : Montepess. (École de méd.) 18 ; s. xiii

Munich : Monacens.   11 ; s. xiv, f. 16
35 ; s. xiii, f. 116 (Liber VII)
13026 (Rat. civ. 26) ; s. xiv, f. 12 (Sine
auctoris nomine)
13054 (Rat. civ. 54)* ; s. xiv, f. 77 (Nic.
Bononiensis expos. super IV.
libros chirurgicales Gal. de ing.
sanit.)

Norfolk : 3443 ; s. —, bibl. Car. Thuyer Cod. Brit. 6605 (Megat.)

Oxford : Coll. Omn. Animar. 68 ; s. xiv, xv, f. 113
Balliol. 213 ; s. xiv in. f. 330 (Expl. duri apostematis
est)
231 ; s. xiv, in. f. 107b (Megat.)
Canonician. (Bodl.) Misc. 504* ; s. xv, f. 131
(abbreviat. Megat.)
Merton. 218 ; s. xiv, f. 1896 (Megat.)
219 ; s. xiv, in. f. 161 (Megat.)
685 ; s. — (Megat.)

Paris : Bibl. de l'Arsenal 1080 ; s. xiv, f. 2ᵛ (abbrev. a Joh.
de St. Amando)
1082 ; s. xvi, f. 1
Bibl. Mazarine 3598 ; s. xiv
Parisin. 6865B ; s. xiv
6883 ; s. xiv, No. 2 (Partic. XIII de m.m. fort
Galeni)

7047* ; s. xv, No. 3 (Ex libr. VII posterior.)
9331 ; s. xv
11860 ; s. xiv, f. 165
14389 ; s. xiv, f. 207
15456 ; s. xiii, f. 61
Nouv. acq. 1482 ; s. —, f. 172 (L. VII–X,
    XIV, partim)

St. Quentin : nr. 107 (94)* ; s. xiv–xv (posterior L. I Johannis
    de Gaddisdon)

Regensburg : Bibl. urb. 45 ; s. — (Sine auctoris nomine)

Rome :   Palat.   1093 ; s. xiv, f. 71 (L. VII–XIV)
             1094 ; s. xiv, f. 115 (De ing. sanit.) et f. 253
                 (Megat.)
             1095 ; s. xiv, f. 3ᵛ (L. VIII–XIV)
             1096 ; s. xiv, f. 14 (L. VII–XIV) et f. 153
                 (L. VII–XIV)
             1097 ; s. —, f. 1
             1098 ; s. xv, f. 33
         Regin.   1305 ; s. —, f. 81
         Urbin.   235 ; s. xiv, f. 1 (Expl. sine flegmone
                 præcedente)
              236 ; s. xiv, f. 1 (L. III–VI, XIII, XIV)
              247 ; s. xiv, f. 205 (L. VII–XIV)
         Vatic.   2375 ; s. xiv, f. 304 et f. 515 (L. VII–XIV)
             2377 ; s. —, f. 1
             2378 ; s. —, f. 1 et f. 121 (Megat.)
             2331 ; s. —, f. 134 (L. VII–XIV)
             2385 ; s. —, f. 187
             2386 ; s. —, f. 145 (L. I, II)
             4421 ; s. —, f. 2 (Libri II)

Venice : Marcian. cl. XIV 6 ; s. xiv, f. 68 (L. VII–XIV)

Würzburg : Bibl. univ. med. f. 2 ; s. xiii ex.

Latin translations

— D. II, f. 101

— C. III, f. 1025 (Thoma Linacro Anglo Interprete)

— Galeni methodus medendi, vel de morbis curandis, T. Linacro . . . interprete. Libri quatuordecim. [Edited by Guillaume Budé.] Lutetiæ. 1519 fol. *540 h. 20 (2)* [B.M.]

— Another copy. With marginal and other corrections of the press in MS. On vellum. Lutetiæ. 1519 fol. *C. 19 e. 17* [B.M.]

Presentation copy to King Henry VIII. The head title is in MS. and is illuminated.

— Another copy, with a dedication to Cardinal Wolsey by Tomas Linacre, and marginal and other corrections of the press in MS. On vellum. Lutetiæ. 1519 fol. *C. 19 e. 16* [B.M.] In this copy the head title is in MS. and is illuminated.

— Another edition. S. Sagnerii index. Parisiis. 1526. 8° *540 d. 3* [B.M.]

— Another edition. Claudii Galeni methodi medendi libri quatuordecim, denuo magna diligentia M. Gregorii recogniti &c. Parisiis, 1538. 8° *541 a. 8* [B.M.]

— Commentarius in sex priores libros Galeni methodi medendi. (With the text of T. Linacre's translation slightly altered). Auctore F. Pacio. Vicetiæ. 1598 fol. *540 h. 17 (1)* [B.M.]

— Commentarius in septimum Galeni librum methodi medendi (with the text) . . . De morbo Gallico per methodum curando, autore F. Pacio. Vicetiæ. 1609 fol. *540 h. 17 (2)* [B.M.]

— Compendium megetechni Galeni a Constantino (Aphricano) compositum. See ISHAK IBN SULAIMAN Ab Israili. Omnia opera Ysaac &c. 1515 fol. *543 h. 1* [B.M.]

— Passionarius Galeni . . . egritudines a capite ad pedes usq. complectens. in quinq. libros particulares, divisus (being an epitome of Galen's books, De Methodo Medendi, with additions from other writers. By Gariopondus). Una cu. febriu. tractu :

earumq. sintomatibus. G. L. Lugduni. 1526. 4° *540 e. 4 (1)* [B.M.]

— Another copy. *46 m. 9* [B.M.]

Methodus medendi—Appendix

— See Caius (J.)   J. Caii de Medendi methodo libri duo ex Claudii Galeni . . . sententia. 1544. 8° *540 d. 7 (4)* [B.M.]

— See Llera (M. de)   D. M. de Llera . . . clavis totius medicinæ . . . speciosora arcana, magisque recondita penitissime expandeus, per octo videlicet libros Methodi Medendi Galeni ; a septimo duntaxat usque ad decimum quartum &c. 1674 fol. *539 k. 15* [B.M.]

— See Maurin (J.)   Quæstio medica . . . An propter motum sanguinis in corde circulatorium mutanda Galeni Methodus Medendi ? 1648.   4° *1182 e. 8 (26)* [B.M.]

— See Reinesius (J. M.)   Commentariolum in Claudii Galeni lib. XIII.   Meth. Med. de ratione curandi Inflammationes &c. 1662.   4° *1179 b. 8 (1)* [B.M.]

— See Sebisch (M.) the Younger.   Collegii therapeutici disputatio I (–XV) continens præcludia in Galeni Methodum Medendi &c. . . . 1634.   4° *1179 i. 3 (3–17)* [B.M.]

(68)

τῶν πρὸς Γλαύκωνα θεραπευτικῶν βιβλία β΄

Ad Glauconem de medendi methodo libri II

Greek, Arabic, and Latin MSS. are known.

Latin MSS.

Angers : Andecavens. 461 (446)* ; s. xvi, f. 67 (Jo. Riolani annotatt.)

Basle : Basil. D I 11 ; s. —

Cesena : Malatest. D XXIII 1 ; s. xiii (De febribus)
                S V 4 ; s. xiv, f. 198

Chartres : Autricens. 62 (115) ; s. x, f. 16 (Des. in 1, I c. 57)
                et f. 38 (Expl. vid. : manifesta
                ratione conscribam)
         Autricens. 293 (351) ; s. xiv, f. 79
Cheltenham : Phillipps. 6915 ; s. xv (De febribus)
Erfurt : Amplon. Q 215 ; s. xiv, f. 102 (Inc. Indigestionem
        abstinentia. Expl. atque fervor nimuetur)
Escurial : Scorial. N III, 17 ; s. xii, f. 41
Glasgow : Hunterian. V, 3, 2 ; s. x (ix), f. — (Expl. in tempore
        suo)
Leipzig : Lipsiens. bibl. univ. Repos. med. I 29 ; s. —
Leyden : Voss. fol. 85 (vide V. Rose præf. ad Theod. Prise.
        p. xv) [2162, 2406]
London : Regius (Br. Mus.) 12 E XX ; s. xii, f. 33
Montecassino : Casinens. 97 ; s. x, f. 33 (Expl. similar to
        Autricens)
Montpellier : Montepess. (École de méd.) 18 ; s. xiii
Munich : Monac. 5 ; s. xiv, f. 112
Paris : Parisin. 6865 ; s. xiv, f. 154c
          nouv. acq. 343 ; s. xiii, f. 55^v (fine mutil.)
Rome : Palat. 1088 ; s. x (?) f. 1 (Initium solum congruit)
          1094 ; s. xiv, f. 525
      Vatic. 2376 ; s. —, f. 213
          2378 ; s. —, f. 48 (Expl. ad Glauconem quæ
             est in prologo de febribus) et f. 105
          2381 ; s. —, f. 221
          2384 ; s. —, f. 57 (Expl. deinceps faciemus
             sermonem)
          4417 ; s. —
          4418 ; s. —
Salamanca : Bibl. univ. 2-4-6 ; s. xvii, No. 2
Upsala : Upsal. C 664 ; s. xi-xii (?), f. 31
Vendôme : Vindocinens. 109 ; s. xi, f. 1 (Expl. dabis libere.
        Explicit liber IV. Galeni)

Latin translations

—   D. II, f. 86

—   C. III, f. 1343 (Nicolao Leoniceno interprete)

—   Galeni de ratione curandi ad Glauconem libri duo.
Interprete N. Acakia.   Ejus-dem interpretis . . . commentarii.
Apud. Juntas : Venetiis, 1547.   8°   *540 c. 12* [B.M.]

—   Another edition.   Lugduni, 1547.   16°   *774 a. 1* [B.M.]

—   Another edition.   Lugduni, 1551.   16°   *540 a. 12* [B.M.]

—   Galeni Pergameni de arte curativa ad Glauconem libri
duo.   (N. Leoniceno interprete.)   Antverpie, 1548.   8°   *540
b. 4 (2)* [B.M.]

—   Stephani Atheniensis . . . explanationes in Galeni priorem
librum Therapeuticum, ad Glauconem.   (With a Latin translation of the text.)   See AKETÆUS.   Medici Antiqui Græci &c.   1581.
4°   *C. 47 f. 15* [B.M.]

—   Explanationes in priorem librum de arte curandi (by V.
Trincavellius).   See Trincavellius, V.

V. Trincavelli in cmnia opera &c.   Tom. 1, pt. 1, 1556 fol.
542 i. 2 [B.M.]

—   Petri Camanes . . . in duos Libros Artis curativæ Galeni
ad Glauconem Commentaria.   (With a Latin translation of the
text.)   Valentiæ, 1625.   4°   *540 f. 11* [B.M.]

De arte curativa—Appendix

—   See Montanus (J. B.)   J. B. Montani . . . in libros Galeni
de arte curandi ad Glauconem explanationes.   1556.   8°   *540
a. 24* [B.M.]

(69)

περὶ φλεβοτομίας πρὸς Ἐρασιστρατείους τοὺς ἐν Ῥώμῃ

De venæ sectione adversus Erasistrateos Romæ degentes

Greek MSS. are known.

Latin translations

— C. III, f. 981 (Inscr. Claud. Galeni De venæ sectione, adversus Erasistratæos, qui Romæ degebant, Liber, Josepho Tectandro Cracoviensi Interprete)

(70)

περὶ φλεβοτομίας πρὸς ᾿Ερασίστρατον

De venæ sectione adversus Erasistratum

Greek MSS. are known.

Latin translations

— C. III, f. 965 (Inscr. C. Galeni De venæ sectione adversus Erasystratum Liber, ad Græcorum exemplarium fidem recognitus, Josepho Tectandro Cracoviensi Interprete)

(71)

περὶ φλεβοτομίας θεραπευτικόν

De curandi ratione per venæ sectionem

Greek and Latin MSS. are known.

Latin MSS.

Dresden : Dresd. Db 92, 93 ; s. xv, f. 319
Paris : Parisin. 6865 ; s. xiv, f. 168

Latin translations

— C. III, f. 1003 (Inscr. C. Galeni De curandi ratione per sanguinis missionem liber, Theodorico Gaudano Interprete)

— Claudii Galeni . . . de curatione per sanguinis missionem libellus. (Commentarius) L. Fuchsio authore. Lugduni, 1546. 8° *774 b. 10 (1)* [B.M.]

— J. N. Rogerii . . . Commentaria in librum Galeni de ratione curandis per sanguinis missionem. (With the text.) Few MS. notes. Campaniæ, 1570. 4° *540 f. 8 (1)* [B.M.]

— Commentaria in librum Galeni de ratione curandi per sanguinis missionem. (With the text.) Auctore H. Nunio Ramirez. Olesipone. 1608. 4° *540 e. 14* [B.M.]

De curandi ratione per venæ sectionem—Appendix

— See SEBISCH (M.) the Younger. Commentarius in libellus Galeni de curandi ratione per sanguinis missionem &c. 1652. 4° *1179 i. 5 (9)* [B.M.]

(72)

περὶ βδελλῶν, ἀντισπάσεως, σικύας καὶ ἐγχαράξεως καὶ κατασχασμοῦ

De hirudinibus, revulsione, cucurbitula, incisione et scarificatione

Greek and Latin MSS. are known.

Latin MSS.

    Madrid : Matrit. bibl. nac. 1978 (ol. L 60) ; s. xiv, f. 118
    Salamanca : Bibl. Univ. 2–4–6 ; s. xvii, No. 4 (Ald Garzeran interprete)

Latin translations

— D. I, f. 149 (Nicolao de Regio interprete)
— C. III, f. 963 (Jano Cornario Medico Physico Interprete)

(73)

περὶ τῆς τῶν καθαιρόντων φαρμάκων δυνάμεως

De purgantium medicamentorum facultate

Greek and Latin MSS. are known.

Latin MSS.

    Cesena : Malatest. D XXIII, 1 ; s. xiii (De simplicibus farmaciis)
                  S. V, 4 ; s. xiv, f. 119 (De simplicibus famarciis)
    Dresden : Dresd. Db 92, 93 ; s. xv, f. 389d
    Paris : Parisin. 6865 ; s. xiv, f. 178a

Rome : Palat. 1094 ; s. xiv, f. 488 (De simplic. farmaciis)
1096 ; s. xiv, f. 124
1098 ; s. xv, f. 16
Urbin. 247 ; s. xiv, f. 67
Vatic. 2378 ; s. —, f. 207
2385 ; s. —, f. 135

Latin translations

— D. I, f. 150

— C. III, f. 303 (Juliano Martiano Rota Interprete)

(74)

τίνας δεῖ ἐκκαθαίρειν καὶ ποίοις καθαρτηρίοις καὶ πότε

Quos, quibus catharticis medicamentis et quando purgare oporteat

Greek and Latin MSS. are known. A Latin MS. is Bernens.
A 91 ; s. xi, f. 4 (Inc. Qui sani sunt corpore in purgationibus.
Expl. si incepta fuerit. amplius provocabitur)

Latin translations

— C. 111, f. 311 (Juliano Martiano Rota Interprete. Inc.
Qui sano corpore . . .)

— Claudii Galeni libellus, cui titulum fecit, quos, quibus
et quando purgare oporteat ; a. S. C. Scipione in linguam
Latinam conversus, ejusdem commentariis illustratus. Cui
accessit materia et forma medicamentorum &c. Lugduni. 1553.
8° *540 a. 25 (2)* [B.M.]

— Another edition. MS. notes. Lugduni, 1557. 8°
540 a. 25 (1) [B.M.]

— Quos, quibus et quando purgare oporteat. See LONICER
(A.) A. Loniceri . . . de Purgationibus libri III. ex . . .
Galeno . . . depromti &c. 1596. 8° *1189 b. 14* [B.M.]

(75)

τῷ ἐπιλήπτῳ παιδὶ ὑποθήκν

Puero epileptico consilium

Greek and Arabian MSS. are known.

Latin translations

— C. III, f. 1487 (Inscr. Claudii Galeni Documentum de Puero Epileptico. Nicolao Leonico Thomæo Patauino Interprete. Argumenta Capitum Consilii pro Puero Epileptico)

(76)

περὶ κράσεως καὶ δυνάμεως τῶν ἁπλῶν φαρμάκων βιβλία ια΄

De simplicium medicamentorum temperamentis et facultatibus libri XI

Greek, Syriac, Arabic, Hebrew, and Latin MSS. are known.

Latin MSS.

Basle : Basil. D III 8 ; s. —

Bordeaux : Burdigalens. 588 ; s. xvi

Breslau : Vratisl. bibl. univ. IV F 25 ; s. xiii, f. 11 (Libri I to V)

Cambrai : Camaracens. 907 (806) ; s. xiv, f. 37

Cambridge : Cantabr. St. Petri 33 ; s. xiii/xiv, f. 131

Cesena : Malatest. D XXIII 1 ; s. xiii (Libri V)

Chartres : Autricens. 384 (340) ; s. xiii, f. 25

Cues : Bibl. Nic. Cusani med. 11 ; s. xiii, xiv, No. 1

Dresden : Dresd. Db 92, 93 ; s. xv, f. 327b (L. I–V) et f. 396b
(L. VI–XI : Secuntur sex ultimi libri de simplici medicina Galieni quo Nicholaus de Regio de greco in latinum transtulit diu post translationem quinque primorum per alium factam)

Erfurt : Amplon. F 249 ; s. xiii, f. 52 (Libri V)

             F 278 ; s. xiv, in. f. 1 (Libri I–VI ?)

             F 280 ; s. xiv, in. f. 1 (L. I–VI) et f. 68 (L. VII–XI)

             Q 178*. ; s. xiii (Inc. Medicina et cibus sunt ambo. Expl. veniat valde perfunde)

Eton : Bibl. Coll. 132 ; s. xiii, No. 12

Leipzig : Lipsiens. bibl. univ. Repos. med. I 29 ; s. —

London : Sloan. 3044 ; s. xvi

Madrid : Matrit. 1198 (ol. L 9) ; s. xiv, f. 74 (Libri V)

             1978 (ol. L 60) ; s. xiv, No. 2

Montpellier : Montepass. (École de méd.) 18 ; s. xiii

Munich : Monac. 11 ; s. xiv, f. 60 (Libri V)

             13054 (Rat. civ. 54)* ; s. xiv, f. 154 (Nicol. Bononiensis Comm.)

Naples : Neapolit. VIII D 34 ; s. xiv (fine mutil.)

Oxford : Coll. Balliol. 231 ; s. xiv, in. f. 283 (Libri V)

        Merton. 218 ; s. xiv, f. 27b (Libri V)

             319 ; s. xiv, in. f. 39 (Libri V)

             685 ; s. —

Paris : Bibl. de l'Arsenal 1080* ; s. xiv, f. 18

             2821* ; s. xvii, f. 90

      Parisin. 6865 ; s. xiv, f. 17 (Libri VI–XI ?)

             11860 ; s. xiv, f. 84

             15456 ; s. xiii, f. 18

             16175 ; s. xiii, f. 19

             nouv. acq. 1482 ; s. —, f. 131

Perugia : Perusin. 44 (A 44) ; s. xv, f. 35–45 (Inc. Et hoc explanat.)

Rome : Palat. 1092 ; s. —, f. 22

             1094 ; s. xiv, f. 31 (L. I–V) et f. 549

             1096 ; s. xiv, f. 101^{v} (L. I–III c. I med; expl. asphaltum et necesse est)

Urbin.   247 ; s. xiv, f. 121 (L. I–V)

         248 ; s. xiv–xv, f. 1

Vatic.   2375 ; s. xiv, f. 27 (L. I–V)

       2376 ; s. —, f. 40 (Libri VI)

       2385 ; s. —, f. 76 (L. I–VI)

       2388 ; s. —, f. 1

       4425* ; s. xiv, f. 204 et 262

St. Gallen : Sangall. 762* ; s. ix, f. 137 (Ex libr. VI. Inc.

           De aloe. Expl. in capite de xirida)

Venice : Marcian. ? (Libri VI)

Latin translations

— D. I, f. 152

— C. III, f. 5 (Theodorico Gaudano Interprete)

— Claudii Galeni . . . de Simplicium medicamentorum facultatibus libri un decim, T. Gerardo . . . interprete. Copious MS. notes. Parisiis, 1530 fol. *539 l. 2 (3)* [B.M.]

— Another edition. Claudii Galeni . . . Libri XI . . . emendatiores exeunt &c. Lugduni, 1561. 8° *774 a. 4* [B.M.]

De simplicium medicamentorum facultatibus—Appendix

— See DANTZE (J.) Tabulæ simplicium medicamentorum quæ apud . . . Galenum . . . sunt &c. 1543 fol. *547 k. 8 (1)* [B.M.]

— See DANTZE (J.) Universales J. Mesue . . . canones . . . una cum quamplurimis ex Galeni libris de simplicium medicamentorum facultatibus &c. 1545 fol. *547 k. 8 (2)* [B.M.]

— See SEBISCH (M.) the Younger. Galeni quinque priores libri de simplicium medicamentorum facultatibus, in sedecim disputationes resoluti &c. 1651 &c. 8° *540 b. 28* [B.M.]

(77)

περὶ συνθέσεως φαρμάκων τῶν κατὰ τόπους βιβλία ι'

De compositione medicamentorum secundum locos libri X

Greek, Arabic, Hebrew, and Latin MSS. are known.

Latin MSS.

Cesena : Malatest. S V 4 ; s. xiv, f. 156 (Inscr. De optima
    compositione medicinarum)

Dresden : Dresd. Db 92, 93 ; s. xv, f. 196a (Inscr. Liber
    Galieni dictus Miamir et aliter decem tractatum
    [f. 256b translatus a Nicholao de Regio . . .
    anno dm MCCCXXXV]

Paris : Bibl. Sainte-Geneviève 1031 ; s. xvii, f. 76 (Anon. comm.)
    Parisin. nouv. acq. 1365 ; s. xiv (Inscr. De passionibus
    unius cuiusque particulæ et cura ipsarum)

Rome : Vatic. 2387 ; s. —, f. 1 (Inscr. similarly to Paris. nouv.
    acq. 1365)

Latin translations

— D. II, f. 158 (Nicolao de Regio interprete)

— C. III, f. 415 (Inscr. Claud. Galeni De compositione
pharmacoru localium, sive secundum locos. Jano Cornario
Medici interprete)

— Claudii Galeni . . . de compositione medicamentorum
secundum locos, seu quæ unicuique corporis parti conveniunt,
libri decem, opus . . . nunc primum Latinitate donatum ac in
lucem æditum per J. Guinterium &c. Parisiis, 1535 fol. *540 l. 9*
[B.M.]

— Universalis doctrina Claudii Galeni . . . de compositione
pharmacorum secundum locos affectos (J. Cornario interprete).
See Actuarius (J.). Compendium ex Actuarii libris de differentiis
urinarum &c. 1541. 8° *540 c. 20* [B.M.]

— Claudii Galeni de compositione pharmacorum localium
libri decem, J. Cornario interprete. Lugduni, 1561. 8° *547 a. 4*
[B.M.]

De compositione medicamentorum secundum locos—Append:x

— See Cornarius (J.) M. D. J. Cornarii . . . in decem
libros Galeni de compositione medicamentorum secundum locos
conscriptos, libri decem &c. 1537 fol. *540 h. 11 (1)* [B.M.]

— See HOLLERIUS (J.) J. Hollerii . . . de morbis internis
lib. II . . . de rhemediis κατὰ τόπους in Galeni libros &c.
1571.   8°   *545 c. 4* [B.M.]

— See Hollerius (J.) J. Hollerii . . . ad libros Galeni
De compositione medicamentorum . . . periochæ VIII. &c.
1589.   8°   *540 a. 27* [B.M.]

(78)

περὶ συνθέσεως φαρμάκων τῶν κατὰ γένη βιβλία ζ′

De compositione medicamentorum per genera libri VII

Greek, Arabic, and Latin MSS. are known.

Latin MSS.

Dresden : Dresd. Db 92, 93* ; s. xv, f. 181a–192c. (Inscr.
        liber catagenarum ; vide Steinschneider :
        Archiv. f. pathol. Anatomice 124 S. 292)

Paris : Parisin. 6865* ; s. xiv, f. 139b–148a (Inscr. the same
        as the Dresden MS.)

Latin translations

— De compositione medicamentorum . . . ex Galeno. See
GESNER (C.) Apparatus et delectus simplicium medicamentorum
&c. 1542.   8°   *1168 e. 7 (1)* [B.M.]

— Claudii Galeni de compositione medicamentorum per
genera libri septem, Joanne (Guinterio) Andernaco interprete.
Nunc denuo . . . castigati . . . ac argumentis et annotationibus
illustrati. Lugduni, 1552.   8°   *540 a. 13* [B.M.]

De compositione medicamentorum per genera—Appendix

— See Rota (J. F.) J. F. Rotæ de introducendis Græcorum
medicaminibus liber. Commentarius sane in Galeni librum
primum de compositione medicamentorum per genera. 1553 fol.
540 h. 11 (2) [B.M.]

(79)

περὶ ἀντιδότων βιβλία δ'

De antidotis libri II

Greek and Arabic MSS. are known.

Latin translations

— C. III, f. 351 (Juliano Martiano Rota interprete)
— De antidotis libri II. A. Lacuna in compendium redacti.
Lat. See EVERARDUS (ÆE.) De herba panacea quam ... Tabacum
... vocant &c. 1587. 8° *549 a. 22* [B.M.]

(80)

πρὸς Πίσωνα περὶ τῆς θηριακῆς

De theriaca ad Pisonem liber

Greek and Arabic MSS. are known.

Latin translations

— C. III, f. 315 (Joanne Andernaco interprete)
— Galeni libellus de Theriaca ad Pisonem ... interprete
J. Jurene. See EVERARDUS (ÆE.) De herba panacea quam ...
Tabacum ... vocant &c. 1587. 8° *549 a. 22* [B.M.]

(81)

περὶ θηριακῆς πρὸς Ταμφιλιανόν

De theriaca ad Pamphilianum

Greek and a Latin MS. are known.

Latin MS.

Cesena : Malatest. S XXVII 4 ; s. xiv, No. 2 (De tyriaca ad
Pamphilum)

Latin translations

— Libellus ad Pamphilianum de Theriaca. Conversus in
Latinum a J. Camerario. See Camerarius (J.) De theriacis

et Mithridateis commentariolus &c. 1550 ? 8° *1038 b. 30 (1)*
[B.M.]

— C. III, f. 345 (Juliano Martiano Rota Interprete) Inscr.
Sed non est genuinus hic Galeni Libellus

(82)

περὶ εὐπορίστων βιβλία γ′

De remediis parabilibus. libri III

Greek and Latin MSS. are known. A Latin MS. is at Rome.
(*Palat. 1298 ; s. —, f. 232.* Inc. Gal. Claudiano Soloni sal.
Quoniam Expl. vel aranea mordicatum.)

Latin translations

— D. II, f. 139 (Nicolao de Regio interprete)

— C. III, f. 1393 (Inscr. Claud. Galeni De remediis paratu
facilibus libellus, ab Huberto Barlando Philiatro Latino Sermoni
traditus, & a Junio Paulo Crasso medico Patauino accuratisime
castigatus)

— C. III, f. 1421 (Inscr. Claudio Galeno Adscriptus Liber de
medicinis facile parabilibus, ad Solonem medicorum principem,
sine principio. Junio Paulo Crasso Patauino Interprete)

— C. III, f. 1455 (Inscr. Liber Tertius de medicamentis,
quæ ad manum, sunt Galeno adscriptus)

— Claudii Galeni de paratu facilibus libellus, H. Barlando
. . . interprete. Antehac neque unquam, neque usquam aut
translatus, aut excusus. Antverpiæ, 1533. 8° *540 d. 1 (1)* [B.M.]

— Liber Galeni de facile acquisibilibus ad Solonem Archi-
medicum ; translatus de greco in latinum a magistro Nicolao de
regio de Calabria. (Book 2 of " De remediis facile parabilibus ".)
See HORTUS. Vitus Sanitatis &c. 1511 fol. *34 f. 8* [B.M.]

— Claudii Galeni . . . de remediis paratu facilibus liber ;
jam olim a Guinterio . . . Latinitate donatus ; nunc autem ex

prelectionibus . . . J. Houllarii . . . repurgatus et . . . illustratus. Paris, 1543. 8° *540 a. 15 (2)* [B.M.]

— Claudii Galeni de remediis parabilibus libellus, omnium rerum capita breviter comprehendens de quibus agitu in decem libris de compositione medicam. Secundum loc., a S. Scrofa in Latinum conversus, multisque in locis castigatus et explicatus. Parisiis, 1548. 8° *540 d. 1 (3)* [B.M.]

(83)

περὶ τῶν παρὰ τὴν λέξιν σοφισμάτων

De captionibus penes dictionem

A single Greek MS. is known.

(84)

περὶ τοῦ προγιγνώσκειν πρὸς Ἐπιγένην

De prægnotione ad Epigenem liber

Greek and Latin MSS. are known.

Latin MSS.

Cesena : Malatest. S V 4 ; s. xiv, f. 130
      S XXVI 4 ; s. xiii, f. 68
Dresden : Dresd. Db 92, 93 ; s. xv, f. 1
Oxford : Coll. S. Joh. Bapt. 17* ; a. 1110, f. 2b
Paris : Parisin. 6865 ; s. xiv, f. 179c

Latin translations

— D. I, f. 272 (Nicolao de Regio interprete)

— C. II, f. 1567 (Inscr. Cl. Galeni de prænotione liber, Jano Cornario Medico Physico interprete. Argumenta capitum quatuordecim libri Galeni de præcognitione, ut Leonardi Jachini translationi inserta sunt)

— Galeni Pergameni de præcognitione libellus, L. Jachino interprete. Ejusdem explanationes in eundem Galeni libellum. Lugduni, 1540. 4° *542 d. 6 (3)* [B.M.]

(85)

εἰσαγωγὴ ἢ ἰατρός

Introductio sive medicus

Greek, Arabic, and Latin MSS. are known.

Latin MSS.

Cesena : Malatest. S V 4 ; s. xiv, f. 42

S XXVI 4 ; s. xiii, f. 35

S XXVII 5 ; s. xiv, No. 1 (Anon. expos. sup. libr. introductoriun Gal.)

Dresden : Dresdens Db. 92, 93 ; s. xv, f. 9a

Florence : Laurent. plut. 73, 9 ; s. xiv, f. 48

Munich : Monacens. 490 ; a. 1488–1503

Paris : Parisin. 6863 [?]

6865 ; s. xiv, f. 2

7030 (?)

7810 ; s. xv

Rome : Palat. 1098 ; s. xv, f. 69

Vatic. 4423 ; s. —, f. 104

Latin translations

— D. I, f. 16

— C. V, Isag. f. 159 (Inscr. Claudio Galeno Adscripta introductio, seu medicus. Quem librum olim Joannes Andernacus fecit ; nuper vero Bartholomæus Sylvanius recognouit ex Græci exemplaris collatione)

(86)

Γαληνοῦ εἰς τὸ Ἱπποκράτους περὶ φύσιος ἀνθρώπου βιβλίον ὑπόμνημα α' β'

Galeni in Hippocratis de natura hominis lib. commentarii II

Greek and Arabic MSS. are known.

Latin translations

— C. I, f. 77 (Hermanno Cruserio Campensi interprete)
— See Hippocrates. De Natura Hominis Claudii Galeni . . .
in Hipp. librum de natura hominis commentarius &c.   1549.   8°
540 a. 7 *(1)* and   — 1570.   8°   *540 a.* 7 *(3)* [B.M.]

(87)

εἰς τὸ περὶ διαίτης ὑγιεινῆς τῶν ἰδιωτῶν Ἱπποκράτους ἢ
Πολύβου ὑπόμνημα

In Hippocratis vel Polybi opus de salubri victus ratione privatorum .
commentarius

Greek and Latin MSS. are known.   A Latin MS. is *Laurent.*
plut. 59. ? ; *s.* —

Latin translations

— C. I, f. 1192 (Inscr. Cl. Galeni In librum de salubri diæta
commentarius, Hermanno Cruserio Campensi interprete)
— See Hippocrates [De victus ratione privatorum] Hippocrates de victus ratione privatorum.   Galeni commentarius
in eundem &c.   1529.   8°   *539 b.* 15 *(2)* [B.M.]

(88)

εἰς τὸ Ἱπποκράτους περὶ τροφῆς ὑπομνήματα δ΄

In Hippocrates librum de alimento commentarii IV

Greek and a Latin MS. are known.

(89)

Ἱπποκράτους περὶ διαίτης ὀξέων νοσημάτων βιβλίον καὶ
Γαληνοῦ ὑυπόμνημα α΄ β΄ γ΄ δ΄

In Hippocratis librum de acutorum victu commentarii IV

Greek, Arabic, Latin, and Hebrew MSS. are known.

Latin MSS.

Brunswick : Bibl. urb. 109 ; s. xiv, f. 184a A

Cambridge : Cantabr. Caius Coll. 59 ; s. xiv (Expl. eis dicat
     ipsas)
    Pembroke. 2055 ; s. —
    St. Petri 14 ; s. xiv, f. 68 (Expl. similar to Caii 59)

Cesena : Malatest. D XXIII 4 ; s. xiv

Chartres : Autricens. 278 (258 et 666) ; s. xiv, f. 132

Cues : Bibl. Nic. Cusani med. 3 ; s. xii, xiii, No. 4
         4 ; s. xii, xiii, No. 4

Erfurt : Amplon. F 246 ; s. xiv, f. 87
     F 255 ; s. xiv, f. 89
     F 264 ; a. 1288, f. 122
     F 266a ; s. xiii ex. f. 62
     F 285 ; a. 1260, f. 87
     F 287 ; s. 1468–71, f. 234
     F 293 ; s. xiii ex. ? f. 169
     Q 178* ; s. xiii (Notulæ huius comm.)

Eton : Bibl. Coll. 127 ; s. xiv, f. 133

Glasgow : Hunterian. T 1. 1 ; s. xiv (Expl. similar to Caii 59)

Laon : Laudunens. 413 ; s. xiv, No. 4
    416 ; s. xiii, No. 6

Leipzig : Lipsiens. bibl. univ. Repos. med. I 22 ; s. —

London : Arundel (Br. Mus.) 162 ; s. xiv, f. 167 (Expl.
    quispiam medicorum)
    Harleian. 5425 ; s. xiii, f. 141

Madrid : Matrit. bibl. nac. 1407 (ol. L 59) ; s. xiv, f. 69
        1408 (ol. L 61) ; s. xv, f. 87

Milan : Ambros. E 78 Inf. ; s. xiv, f. 62

Munich : Monac. 31 ; a. 1302, f. 80
     187 ; s. xiii, f. 220
     270 ; s. xiv, f. 73
     3512 (Aug. civ. 12) ; a. 1300, f. 403 (Comm.
     in Hipp. particular III)

Naples : Neapolit. VIII D 25 bis ; s. xiv, f. 122
Oxford : Coll. Omn. Animar. 68 ; s. xiv, xv, f. 63
                              71 ; s. xiv in. f. 87 (Inc. mutil).
                                 (Et scias quod victus hore)
         St. Joh. Bapt. 10 ; s. xiii ex. f. 61
         Merton. 220 ; s. xiv, f. 78 (Expl. similar to Caii 59)
                   221 ; s. xiv, f. 103b (Expl. de quibus
                        deinceps faciam sermonem)
                   687
                   689
         Novi   170 ; s. xiv, f. 206b
                   1130
                   1134
         Univ.   89 ; s. xv in. f. 203 (Inc. partis huius artis)
Paris : Parisin.   7030A ; s. xiv, No. 7
                   16174 ; s. xiii, f. 81
                   16177 ; s. xiii ex. f. 249 (sine auctoris nomine)
                   16188 ; s. xiii, f. 140
                   17157 ; s. xiv, f. 97
                   18500 ; s. xiii ex. f. 72
                   Nouv. acq. 1480 ; s. xiv, f. 211
                              1481 ; s. xiv, f. 70
Pavia : Bibl. Univ. 383 ; s. xv, f. 47
Rome :   Ottobonian. 1158 A ; s. —, f. 63
         Palat. 1102 ; s. —, f. 83
                   1103 ; s. —, f. 145
         Regin. 1270 ; s. xiv, f. 160
                   1302 ; s. xiv, f. 160
         Vatic. 2390 ; s. —, f. 23
                   2391 ; s. —, f. 127
                   2392 ; s. —, f. 35
                   2393 ; s. —, f. 49
                   2394 ; s. —, f. 109
                   2395 ; s. —, f. 75

2417 ; s. —, f. 96 (in partic. IV)
2428 ; s. —, f. 136
4419 ; s. —, f 135 (imperf.)
4420 ; s. —, f. 23

St. Gallen : Vadian. 431 ; a. 1465

Upsala: Upsal. C 661; s. xiii, f. 273 (Inc. Cum de ægrotantium accidentibus. Expl. similar to Caii 59)

Utrecht : Traiectan. Bibl. univ. 679 ; s. xiv, in. f. 30–73

Latin translations

— C. IV, f. 5 (Joanne Vasseo Meldensi Interprete) Inc. Qui Guidias appellatas sententias conscripserut. Expl. de quibus deinceps faciá sermonem.

(90)

τῶν εἰς τὸ περὶ χυμῶν Ἱπποκράτους ὑπομνημάτων τὸ α′ β′ γ′

In Hippocratis de humoribus librum commentarii III

The Greek MSS. are known. This work is shown in the Index Catalogue of the British Museum, as a supposititious work of Galen.

Latin translations

— See Hippocrates. Ἱπποκράτους περὶ χυμῶν. Hippocratis liber de humoribus . . . Galeni in eundem librum commentarius &c. Greek and Latin. 1555. 4° *539 g. 27 (2)* [B.M.]

— A Piccolhomini . . . in librum Galeni de humoribus commentarii (with the text). Greek & Latin. Aldus, Parisiis. 1556. 8° *7440 a. 11* [B.M.]

— Another copy. *540 d. 17* [B.M.]

Imperfect : wanting two folding leaves of tables.

— Galeni de humoribus liber . . . nunc primum ex Græco in Latinum sermonem . . . conversus, a B. Bertrando . . . Hinc ab eodem interprete insertæ sunt in ipso margine utiles annotationes &c. Greek & Latin. Argentorati. 1558. 8° *540 b. 15 (2)* [B.M.]

(91)

εἰς τὸ Ἱπποκράτους προρρητικῶν βιβλίον πρῶτον ὑπόμνημα
α′ β′ γ′

In Hippocratis prædictionum librum primum commentarii III

Greek and Latin MSS. are known. A Latin MS. is at Rome
(Reg. Suec. 947 ; s. —)

Latin translations

— See Hippocrates. 1526 which contains "Prædictiones
cum Galeni commentariis". *539 d. 7* [B.M.]

— See Hippocrates . . . Prædictiones Hippocratis cum
Galeni commentarii &c. . . . 1537. 8° *549 a. 6* [B.M.]

(92)

Ἱπποκράτους: εἰς—ἐπιδημίας

In Hippocratis epidemiarum libros

Ἱπποκράτους ἐπιδημιῶν α′ καὶ Γαληνοῦ εἰς αὐτὸ ὑπόμνημα
α′ β′ γ′

In Hippocratis epidemiarum librum primum commentarii III

Ἱππ ἐπιδ. β′ καὶ Γ. εἰς αὐτὸ ὑπ. α′ β′ γ′ δ′ ε′

In librum secundum commentarii V

Ἱππ. ἐπιδ. γ′ καὶ Γ. εἰς αὐτὸ ὑπ. α′ β ′γ′

In librum tertium commentarii III

Ἱππ. ἐπιδ. ζ′ καὶ Γ. εἰς αὐτὸ ὑπ. α′ β′ γ′ δ′ ε′ ζ

In librum sextum commentarii VI

In lib. I : Inc. (lib. 1) οὐκ ἐν τούτῳ μὲν βιβλίῳ Ἱπποκράτης
   Expl. (lib. 3) ἡ γυνὴ διὰ τὴν ἰσχὺν τῆς φύσεως
     σωθῆναι

In lib. II : Inc. (lib. 1) ἄνθρακες ἐν κρανῶνι
   Expl. (lib. 5) αἷμα συλλέγεται αἰτῷ ἐπὶ τοὺς τιτθοὺς

In lib. III : Inc. (lib. 1) πυθίων ὃς ᾤκει παρὰ γῆς ἱερόν

Expl. (lib. 3) εἰδέναι οὓς καὶ ὅτε καὶ ὡς δεῖ διαιτᾶν

In lib. VI : Inc. (lib. 1) ἐλυμήναντο πολλοὶ τῶν ἐξηγηῖῶν

Expl. (lib. 6) ποδάγρας τε καὶ ἀρθριτίδας

Of the MSS., the Greek, Latin, and Arabic are known.

Latin MSS.

Erfurt : Amplon. Q 201 ; s. xiv in. (Sub nomine Joannis
Alexandrini, qui Gal. opus transtulit ; in librum VI.
Inc. Quoniam determinant Hipp. de acutis. Expl.
multa fecimus et nihil profecismus)

Rome : Regin. 1305 ; s. —, f. 1 (Similar to Amplon. Inc.
Post. quan.)

Vatic. 2396 ; s. xvi, f. 1 (Inc. Gal. in primum epidem.
Hipp. Expl. partibus interioribus
abdominis)

Latin translations

— See Hippocrates. De Epidemiis. Libri epidemiorum
Hippocratis primus, tertius, et sextus, cum Galeni in eos commentariis &c. 1550. 8° 774 a. 9 [B.M.]

In Hippocratis de Epidemiis Libros—Greek & Latin

— Claudii Galeni Commentarius in secundum Epidemiorum
Hippocratis . . . e Græco . . . translatus a J. SOZOMENO (Pars
secunda—tertia). Greek & Latin. Venetiis. 1617. 8° 540 b. 7
[B.M.]

(93)

Ἱπποκράτους ἀφορισμοὶ καὶ Γαληνοῦ εἰς αὐτοὺς ὑπομνήματα ζ'

Hippocratis aphorismi et Galeni in eos commentarii VII

Greek, Arabic, Latin, and Hebrew MSS. are known.

Latin MSS.

Autun : Augustodun. 70 ; s. xiv, No. 1

Breslau : Vratisl. bibl. acad. Aa IV F 24 ; s. xv, f. 1–119a

Brussels : Bruxell. 14301–14305 ; s. —, No. 111 (Inc. Corpora
  non quis)

Cambridge : Cantabr. St. Petri   14 ; s. xiv, f. 1
  186 ; s. —

Chartres : Autricens. 286 (342) ; s. xiv, f. 17

Copenhagen : Bibl. reg. Thottian. 189 : s. xiv, f. 3

Cues : Bibl. Nic. Cusani med. 4 ; s. xii, xiii, No. 1

Erfurt : Amplon. F 246 ; s. xiv, f. 1
  F 255 ; s. xiv, f. 10
  F 264 ; a. 1288, f. 90
  F 266a ; s. xiii ex. f. 1
  F 285 ; a. 1260, f. 15
  F 287 ; a. 1468–71, f. 55
  F 293 ; s. xiii ex. ? f. 1
  Q 178 ; s. xiii, f. 57

Eton : Bibl. Coll. 127 ; s. xiv, f. 22

Glasgow : Hunterian. T. 1. 1 ; s. xiv

Laon : Laudunens. 413 ; s. xiv, No. 1
  416 ; s. xiii, No. 4

Leipzig : Lipsiens. bibl. univ. Repos. med. I 22 ; s. —
  I 28 ; s. —

London : Arundel. 162 ; s. xiv, f. 115

Madrid : Matrit. bibl. nac. 1407 (ol. L 59) ; s. xiv, f. 3
  1408 (ol. L 61) ; s. xv, f. 12

Milan : Ambros. E 78 Inf. ; s. xiv, f. 5

Metz : Mediomatric. 174 ; s. xiv, No. 2
  177 ; s. xiv, No. 6

Montpellier : Montepess. (École de méd.) 186 ; s. xiv, No. 3

Munich : Monac.   31.; a. 1320, f. 1

                  161 ; s. xiii, f. 41 (Aph. ad chirurg.
                      pertinentes)

                  168 ; s. xiv, f. 23

                  187 ; s. xiii, f. 8

                  270 ; s. xiv, f. 10

                  3512 (Aug. civ. 12) ; a. 1300, f. 340

                  13034 (Rat. civ. 34) ; s. xiv, f. 49

Naples : Neapolot. VIII D 25 ; a. 1380

                 VIII D 25 bis ; s. xiv, f. 1

                 VIII D 38 ; s. xiv, f. 78

Nürnberg : Ebnerian. fol. 129 ; s. xiii, No. 4 (Comm. in libr.
        I et II)

Oxford : Coll. Omn. Animar. 68 ; s. xiv, xv, f. 1

                        71 ; s. xiv, in. f. 13

        Coll. St. Joh. Bapt. 10 ; s. xiii ex. f. 1

        Coll. Merton. 220 ; s. xiv, f. 39

                221 ; s. xiv, f. 19

                222 ; s. xiv, f. 94

                689 ; s. —

        Novi 1134 ; s. —

Padua : Bibl. Joannis Rhodii (whereabouts not known)

Paris : Parisin.   6846 ; s. xiv

             6860A ; s. xiv, No. 2

             6869 ; s. xiv, No. 4

             6870 ; s. xiv, No. 5

             6871 ; s. xiv, No. 4

             7030A ; s. xiv, No. 5

           15457 ; s. xiii ex. f. 116

           16174 ; s. xiii, f. 1

           16177 ; s. xiii ex. f. 15

           16178 ; s. xiv, f. 11

           17157 ; s. xiv, f. 17

           18500 ; s. xiii ex. f. 107

Nouv. acq. 1480 ; s. xiv, f. 144

1481 ; s. xiv, f. 42 (Finis tantum)

St. Gallen : Vadian. 431 ; a. 1463, f. 3

St. Quentin : nr. 104 (91) ; s. xiii, No. 2

Ste. Giatiani : Turonens. 395 Montf. 11 1277. Cath. Metens.

Ap. Montf.

Regensburg : Bibl. urb. 70 ; s. —

Rome : Ottobon. 1158 A ; s. —, f. 1 et 88

Palat.   1089 ; s. —, f. 27

1102 ; s. —, f. 15

1103 ; s. —, f. 11

1104 ; s. —, f. 3

1196 ; s. —, f. 11

Regin.   396 ; s. —

1270 ; s. xv, f. 1

1302 ; s. xiv, f. 1

Vatic.   2366 ; s. xiv–xv, f. 3

2367 ; s. xiv, f. 1

2368 ; s. —, f. 3

2369 ; s. —, f. 1

2390 ; s. —, f. 1

2391 ; s. —, f. 1

2392 ; s. —, f. 1

2393 ; s. —, f. 1

2394 ; s. —, f. 1

2395 ; s. —, f. 1

2417 ; s. —, f. 17

2428 ; s. —, f. 63

4419 ; s. —, f. 30

4420 ; s. —, f. 57

4439 ; s. —, f. 42

Turin : Taurin. ap. Montf. 11 1398

Upsala : Upsal. C 661 ; s. xiii, f. 1

Utrecht : Traiectan. Bibl. Univ. 679; s. xiv in. f. 1. (c. lacunis)

Venice : Marcian. App. cl. XIV 3 ; s. xvi (Matth. Curcii expos.
in 1. 11. aph. c expos. Galeni)
Wolfenbüttel : Guerferbyt. 2194 (17.2. Aug.) ; a. 1444, f. 1–93

Latin translations

— C. IV, f. 535 (Nicolao Leoniceno Interprete, a Martiano
Rota, & a Jano Cornario diligentissime recogniti)

— Liber aphorismorum [of Hippocrates with Galen's
commentary]. See HUNAIN IBN ISHAK. Begin. In hoc pclaro
libro sut. ista opa. &c. 1487 fol. *540 k. 15* [B.M.]

— Hippocratis Aphorismi cum commento Galeni. See
ARTICELLA. Artesela 1491 fol. *I. B. 23620* [B.M.]

— See Hippocrates. Aphorismi. *Begin*. Laurentii Laurentiani . . . in Sententias Hippocratis præfatio &c. *End*. Finiunt
Sententiæ Hippocratis et item commentationes Galeni in eas
ipsas sententias &c. 1494 fol. *I. B. 27225* [B.M.]

— See Hippocrates. Aphorismi. Expositio Ugonis Senensis
super aphorismos Hypocratis, super commentum Galeni ejus
interpretis &c. [With a Latin version of the text of both authors.]
1498 fol. *I. B. 22979* [B.M.]

— See Hippocrates. Aphorismi. Habes in hoc volumine . . .
particulas septem Apho. Hyppo. . . . cum expositionibus magni
Galeni &c. 1508 fol. *539 i. 4 (1)* [B.M.]

— See Hippocrates. Aphorismi. Expositio Ugonis Senensis
super Aforismos Hippocratis : super commentum Galeni ejus
interpretis. [With the text of both authors in Latin.] 1517 fol.
7305 g. 19 [B.M.]

— See Hippocrates. Aphorismi. Jacobus de Forlivio super
afforismis . . . una cum Galeni . . . commentariis &c. 1520
fol. *537 i. 5 (1)* [B.M.]

— See Hippocrates. Two or more works. Latin. Hippocratis . . . Aphorismorum et sententiarum libri septem (quibus
apposita est . . . enarratio . . . Galeni aut Oribasii aut . . .
utriusque mixta) &c. 1537 4° *539 e. 15 (1)* [B.M.]

— Galeni . . . in Aphorismos Hippocratis liber primus (–septimus) Nicolao Leoniceno . . . interprete.

See Hippocrates. Aphorismi. A. M. Brasavoli in octo libros aphorismorum Hippocratis et G. commentaria &c. 1541 fol. *339 i. 6* [B.M.]

— See Hippocrates. Aphorismi. Donati a Mutiis . . . in interpretationem Galeni super quatuordecim aphorismos Hippocratis dialogus. 1547. 4° *540 e. 7 (2)* [B.M.]

— See Hippocrates. Aphorismi. Claudii Galeni in aphorismos Hippocratis commentaria &c. 1633. 12° *540 a. 19* [B.M.]

Greek & Latin

— See Hippocrates. Aphorismi. Galeni in Aphorismos Hippocratis commentarii septem &c. Greek & Latin. 1532. 8° *540 d. 15* [B.M.]

— See Hippocrates. Aphorismi Hippocratis Aphorismorum genuina lectio . . . Eorundem . . . interpretatio cum Galeni censura &c. Greek & Latin. 1547. 8° *539 c. 2 (1)* [B.M.]

— See Hippocrates. Aphorismi. Aphorismi Hippocratis . . . una cum Galeni commentariis &c. Greek & Latin. 1549. 8° *774 a. 7* [B.M.]

— See Hippocrates. Aphorismi. Hippocratis Aphorismi . . . Galeni in eosdem commentarii septem &c. Greek & Latin. 1561. 8° *774 a. 8* [B.M.]

— See Hippocrates. Aphorismi. Hippocratis Aphorismi . . . Galeni in eosdem commentarii septem . . . J. Marinelli commentarii in Aphor. qui cum Galeni commentariis æquo animo conferantur. Greek & Latin. 1582. 8° *540 a. 18* [B.M.]

— See Hippocrates. Aphorismi. Aphorismi Hippocratis . . . una cum Galeni commentariis &c. Greek & Latin. 1668. 16° *540 a. 20* [B.M.]

In Hippocratis aphorismos commentarius—Appendix

— See Hippocrates. Aphorismi. Hippocratis . . . aphorismorum sectiones septem . . . adjectis annotationibus, in quibus

quotquot sunt in Galeni commentariis loci difficiles, ad unguem
explicantur. Greek & Latin. 1545. 8° *539 d. 17* [B.M.]
— See Hippocrates Aphorismi. Hippocratis aphorismi ex
nova Claudii Campensii . . . interpretatione. Ejus-dem in
aphorismos annotationes, quibus illustrantur evidentissima Galeni
errata. His deinde nexæ sunt animadversiones simul cum
apologia in Galenum &c. Greek & Latin. 1579. 8° *539 c. 10 (2)*.
[B.M.]
— See Benzo (U.) Senensis. Ugo Senensis super aphorismos
Hypo. sup. cometu. Gal. ejus interpretis. 1493 fol. *I. B. 25743*
[B.M.]

(94)

πρὸς λύκον

Adversus Lycum

The Greek MSS. are known.

Latin translations

— C. IV, f. 759 (Julio Alexandrino Tridentino Interprete)

(95)

πρὸς τὰ ἀντειρημένα τοῖς Ἱπποκράτους ἀφορισμοῖς ὑκὸ
Ἰουλιάνου βιβλίον

*Adversus ea quæ a Juliano in Hippocratis aphorismos enuntiata
sunt libellus*

The Greek MSS. are known.

Latin translations

— C. IV, f. 759 (Julio Alexandrino Tridentino Interprete)

(96)

Ἱπποκράτους τὸ περὶ ἄρθρων βιβλίον καὶ Γαληνοῦ εἰς αὐτὸ
ὑπομνήματα δ´

In Hippocratis de articulis librum commentarii IV

Greek MSS. are known.

Latin translations

— C. IV, f. 345 (Joanne Bernardo Feliciano Interprete)
— Liber Hippocratis de articulis, cum IIII. Galeni commentariis. See Vidius (V.) the Elder. Chirurgia &c. 1544 fol. *545 1. 7* [B.M.]

In Hippocratis de articulis librum—Appendix

— See TRILLER (D. W.) Ordinis medici . . . Decanus D.W. Trillerus . . . panegyrici . . . indicit, præmisa exercitatione de macie corporis . . . ad quendam Galeni locum (Comment. I. in Hippocrat. Lib. de articulis Text XXIX, page 208) &c. 1772. 4° *7306 e. 14 (12)* [B.M.]

(97)

περὶ τῶν ἐπιδέσμων

De fasciis

Greek and Latin MSS. are known. A Latin MS. is Parisin 6866 ; s. xvi, No. 4

Latin translations

— C. IV, f. 503 (anon. interpr.)
— Liber Galeni de fasciis. [Translated by V. Vidius.] See Vidius (V.) the Elder. Chirurgia &c. 1544 fol. *545 1. 7* [B.M.]
— Galeni . . . de fasciis libellus a V. Vidio . . . Latinitate donatus congruisque iconibus illustratus. Lyons, 1553 ? 8° *774 a. 5 (2)* [B.M.]
— Another edition. See GESNER (C.). De Chirurgia scriptores optimi &c. 1555 fol. *42 h. 8* [B.M.]

(98)

Ἱπποκράτους προγνωστικὸν καὶ Γαληνοῦ εἰς αὐτὸ ὑπόμνημα ά β' γ'

In Hippocratis prognosticum commentarii III

Greek, Arabic, Latin and Hebrew MSS. are known.

Latin MSS.

Autun : Augustodun. 70 ; s. xiv, No. 2

Brussels : Bruxell. 14301–14305 ; s. —, No. iv

Cambridge : Cantabr. Caius Coll. 57 ; s. xiv, f. 59

                             954 ; s. —

           St. Petri 14 ; s. xiv, f. 41

           Univ. J i 11 5 ; s. xiv, f. 41 (in libr. I et II capp. 46. Expl. et ego quidem iam ostendi in alio)

Chartres : Autricens. 278 (258 et 666) ; s. xiv, f. 106

                  286 (342) ; s. xiv, f. 110

Copenhagen : Bibl. reg. Thottian. 189 ; s. xiv, f. 39

Cues : Bibl. Nic. Cusani med. 3 ; s. xii, xiii, No. 2

                            4 ; s. xii, xiii, No. 2

                            6 ; s. xiii/xiv, No. 1

Erfurt : Amplon. F 246 ; s. xiv, f. 53

                F 255 ; s. xiv, f. 56

                F 264 ; a. 1288, f. 150

                F 266 ; s. xiii ex. f. 38

                F 285 ; a. 1260, f. 58

                F 287 ; a. 1468–71, f. 114

                F 293 ; s. xiii ex. ? f. 53

Eton : Bibl. Coll. 127 ; s. xiv, f. 87

Glasgow : Hunterian. T. 1. 1 ; s. xiv

Laon : Laudunens. 413 ; s. xiv, No. 2

                416 ; s. xiii, No. 5

Leipzig : Lipsiens. bibl. univ. Repos. med. I 22 ; s. —

                                I 28 ; s. —

London : Arundel. 162 ; s. xiv, f. 9

Madrid : Matrit. bibl. nac. 1407 (ol. L 59) ; s. xiv, f. 43

                     1408 (ol. L 61) ; s. xv, f. 55

Metz : Mediomatric. 177 ; s. xiv, No. 7

Montpellier : Montepess. (École de méd.) 188 ; s. xiv, No. 4

Munich : Monac. 31 ; a. 1302, f. 47

            168 ; s. xiv, f. 88

            187 ; s. xiii, f. 171

            270 ; s. xiv, f. 44

            3512 (Aug. civ. 12) ; a. 1300, f. 378

Naples : Neapolit. VIII D 25 ; a. 1380

            VIII D 25 bis ; s. xiv, f. 74

Nürnberg : Ebnerian. fol. 129 ; s. xiii, No. 4

Oxford : Coll. Omn. Animar. 68 ; s. xiv, xv, f. 45

                       71 ; s. xiv in. f. 646

      Bodl. 439 ; s. —

      Canonic. (Bodl.) 272 ; s. xiv ex. f. 57

      Coll. S. Joh. Bapt. 10 ; s. xiii ex. f. 37

      Coll. Merton. 220 ; s. xiv, f. 30

               221 ; s. xiv, f. 69b

               222 ; s. xiv, f. 146b

      Coll. Novi. 170 ; s. xv, f. 162

      Coll. Univ. 89 ; s. xiv in. f. 155 (Initio mutil.)

Paris : Parisin. 6846 ; s. xiv (Initio mutil.)

            6860A ; s. xiv, No. 1 (Comm. qui bidetur

                excesse e Gal.)

            15457 ; s. xiii, f. 88

            16174 ; s. xiii, f. 49

            16177 ; s. xiii ex. f. 197

            16178 ; s. xiv, f. 41

            16188 ; s. xiii, f. 94

            17157 ; s. xiv, f. 63

            18500 ; s. xiii ex. f. 131

            nouv. acq. 1480 ; s. xiv, f. 17

                   1481 ; s. xiv, f. 43

      Bibl. Univ. 580 ; s. xiv

Regensburg : Bibl. urb. 71 ; s. —
Rome : Ottobon. 1158A ; s. —, f. 41
        Palat.   1102 ; s. —, f. 32
                  1103 ; s. —, f. 57
                  1104 ; s. —, f. 34
Rome : Regin.   396 ; s. —
                   974 ; s. —
                  1270 ; s. xiv, f. 124
                  1302 ; s. xiv, f. 123
        Vatic.   2368 ; s. xiv–xv, f. 30
                  2390 ; s. —, f. 59
                  2391 ; s. —, f. 97
                  2392 ; s. —, f. 58
                  2393 ; s. —, f. 30
                  2394 ; s. —, f. 66
                  2395 ; s. —, f. 45
                  2417 ; s. —, f. 62
                  2428 ; s. —, f. 109
                  4419 ; s. —, f. 1 (Init. et fine mutil.)
                  4420 ; s. —, f. 1
St. Gall. : Vadian. 431 ; a. 1465
Upsala : Upsal. C 661 ; s. xiii, f. 207
Wolfenbüttel : Guerferbyt. 2194 (17. 2 Aug.) ; a. 1444,
                f. 99ᵛ–110 (in partes II et III)
                Cathedr. Metens. 229 ap. Montf. II 1386

Latin translations

— C. II, f. 1475 (Laurentio Laurentiano Florentino Interprete)
— Liber pnosticor. [of Hippocrates with Galen's commentary]. See HUNAIN IBN ISHAK. Begin : In hoc polaro libro sut ista opa &c. 1487 fol. *540 k. 15* [B.M.]
— See Hippocrates. [Prognostica] Contenta. Prædictiones sive prognostica Hippocratis . . . Claudii Galeni commentarii in eosde . . . Laurentiano interprete. 1516 fol. *539 h. 5 (1)* [B.M.]

— See Hippocrates. [Prognostica] Liber prognosticorum Hippocratis . . . additis annotationibus in Galeni commentarios &c. 1552 fol. *539 h. 10* [B.M.]

— See Hippocrates (Prognostica] Claudii Galeni in Hippocr. . . . prognosticum commentarius in treis libros divisus &c. 1552. 8° *774 a. 10 (1)* [B.M.]

— V. Trincavelli in primam partem secundi lib. Prognostic. Hippoc. et Gal. familiares exercitationes. [With the text interpolated by V. Trincavellius.] See Trincavellius, V. V. Trincavellii . . . omnia opera &c. Tom. 2 part 1. 1586 fol. *542 i. 2* [B.M.]

In Hippocratis Prognostica—Greek & Latin

— See Hippocrates. [Prognostica] Ἱπποκράτους κώου προγνωστικῶν βίβλοι γ' . . . Cum Claudii Galeni tribus in eosdem commentariis &c. Greek & Latin. 1543. 8° *539 d. 28 (2)* [B.M.]

— See Hippocrates. [Prognostica] Ἱπποκράτους . . . προγνωστικά . . . Latina ecphrasis ex mente Galeni &c. Greek & Latin. 1575. 8° *539 g. 27 (3)* [B.M.]

(99)

εἰς τὸ Ἱπποκράτους περὶ ἀγμῶν ὑπόμνημα ά β' γ'

In Hippocratis librum de fracturis commentarii III

Greek and Latin MSS. are known.

Latin MSS.

Paris : Parisin. 6861 ; s. xvi
      6866 ; s. xvi No. 1

Latin translations

— C. IV, f. 245 (Joanne Bernardo Feliciano Interprete)

(100)

τὸ 'Ιπποκράτους κατ' ἰητρεῖον βιβλίον καὶ Γαληνοῦ εἰς αὐτὸ
ὑπόμνημα καὶ Γαληνοῦ εἰς αὐτὸ ὑπόμνημα ά β' γ'

In Hippocratis librum de officina medici commentarii III

Greek MSS. are known.

Latin translations

— Liber Hippocratis de Officina Medici cu. III.   Galen
commentariis.   See Vidius V. the Elder.   Chirurgia &c.   1544 fol.
545 1. 7 [B.M.]

(101)

περὶ μυῶν ἀνατομῆς

De musculorum dissectione

Greek and Arabic MSS. are known.

(102)

πῶς δεῖ ἐξελέγχειν τοὺς προσποιουμένους νοσεῖν

Quomodo morbum simulantes sint deprehendendi

Greek and Latin MSS. are known.

Latin MSS.

Cesena : Malatest. S V 4 ; s. xiv, f. 37
                        S XXVI 4 ; s. xiii, f. 25
Dresden : Dresd. Db 92. 93 ; s. xv, f. 19a
Erfurt : Amplon. F 236 ; s. xiv
Munich : Monacens. 490 ; a. 1488–1503
Paris : Parisin. 6865 ; s. xiv, f. 117a
Rome : Palat. 1098 ; s. xv, f. 7
            Vatic. 2378 ; s. —, f. 120

Latin translations

— D. II, f. 1
— C. V, Isag. f. 195 (Joanne Fichardo Francofordiano olim
interprete, nunc vero locis in eo compluribus ex Græci codicis
fide restitutis)

(103)

περὶ τῶν ἰδίων βιβλίων

De libris propriis

A Greek MS. survives at Milan.

Latin translations

— C. V, Isag. f. 33 (Joanne Fichardo Francofordiano
Latinitate Donatus)

— Galeni de propriis libris liber. See Caius J. J. Caii
opera aliquot et versiones. 1556. 8° *246 k. 6* [B.M.]

(104)

περὶ τῆς τάξεως τῶν ἰδίων βιβλίων πρὸς Εὐγενιανόν

De ordine librorum suorum ad Eugenianum

Known in Greek manuscript.

Latin translations

— C. V, Isag. f. 47 (A Joanne Fichardo Francofordiano olim
Latinitate donatus)

— Galeni de ordine librorum suroum liber. See CAIUS (J.)
J. Caii . . . opera aliquot et versiones. 1556. 8° *246 k. 6*
[B.M.]

De ordine librorum suroum—Greek & Latin

— Regiæ . . . literarum Universitatis Prorector A. Bech-
mann. . . . Successorem suum civibus academicii commendat.
Galeni libellum qui inscribitur περὶ τῆς τάξεως τῶν ἰδίων βιβλίων
recensuit et explanavit Iwanus Nueller. Greek and Latin.
Erlangæ. 1874. 4° *7320 f. 16* [B.M.]

(105)

τῶν Ἱπποκράτους γλωσσῶν ἐξήγησις

Linguarum s. dictionum exoletarum Hippocratis explicatio

The Greek MSS. are known.

Latin translations

— C. IV, f. 777 (Inscr. Claudii Galeni obsoletarum Hippocratis vocum, Expositio, Jano Cornario Medico Physico Interprete)

— Hippocratis vocum explanationes . . . Galeni &c. See Hippocrates—Works. Hippocratis opera quæ extant &c. Greek and Latin. 1588 fol. *539 i. 3* [B.M.]

— Galeni obsoletarum Hippocratis vocum explanationes Græco latinæ. See Erotian. Erotiani, Galeni et Herodoti Glossaria in Hippocratem &c. 1780. 8° *1090 1. 2* [B.M.]

(106)

εἰ ζῷον τὸ κατὰ γαστρός

An animal sit quod est in utero

Greek MSS. are known.

Latin translations

— C. I, f. 1025 (Inscr. Cl. Galeni Liber falso adscriptus An animal sit id, quod in utero est. Horatio Limano Interprete)

— Claudii Galeni Pergameni utrum conceptus in utero sit animal, M. T. Melanelio . . . interprete. Antverpiæ, 1540. 4° *540 e. 11 (1)* [B.M.]

(107)

περὶ τῆς κατὰ τὸν Ἱπποκράτην διαίτης ἐπὶ τῶν ὀξέων νοσημάτων

De victus ratione in morbis acutis ex Hippocratis sententia

Greek MSS. are known.

Latin translations

— C. IV, f. 5 (Inscr. Claud. Galeni in Librum Hippocratis De Victus Ratione in Morbis acutis . . . Joanne Vassæo Meldensi Interprete)

— See Hippocrates. [De victus ratione in morbis acutis] Galeni in librum Hippocratis de victus ratione in morbis acutis

commentarii quatuor, J. Vassæo interprete &c. 1531 fol.
539 1.2 (1) [B.M.]

— 1542. 8° *540 d. 13* [B.M.]

— See Hippocrates [De victus ratione in morbis acutis]
'Ιπποκράτους . . . τὸ περὶ διαίτης ὀξέων νοσημάτον, De victus
ratione . . . una cum Galeni quatuor in eundem commentariis,
J. Vassæo interprete &c. 1543. 8° *540 d. 14* [B.M.]

— 1546 fol. *539 h. 8* [B.M.]

— 1563. 8° *540 a. 33 (2)* [B.M.]

— See Hippocrates. [De victus ratione in morbis acutis]
Hippocratis de victu acutorum sive de ptissana libri tres, et
Galeni commentaria, Nicolao Lavachio interprete &c. 1533. 4°
539 e. 6 [B.M.]

(108)

περὶ φιλοσόφου ἱστορίας

De historia philosophia

Greek and Latin MSS. are known. A Latin MS. is Monacens.
465 ; a. 1503, f. 53 (Apogr. libri Venetiis a, 1503 editi)

Latin translations

— C. IV, f. 803 (Inscr. Claudii Galeni Liber De Historia
Philosophica, Jano Martiano Rota Interprete)

(109)

ὅροι ἰατρικοί

Definitiones medicæ

Greek and Latin MSS. are known. This work is described as
one of the " Supposititious Works " of Galen, in the Index
Catalogue of the British Museum.

Latin MSS.

Florence : Laurent. plut. 73, 9 ; s. xvi, f. 5 (Euphrosyno
Bonino interprete)

Rome : Vatic. 4423 ; s. —, f. 1 (Euphrosyno Bonino interprete)

Gal. de definitionibus est, ut puto latine, inter MSS. bibl. Jacobeæ n. 8484 (Achermann's *Hist. litteraria* Hoppocratis)

Latin translations

— C. V, Isag. f. 135 (Inscr. Claud. Galeno Adscriptæ Finitiones Medicæ, Bartholomæo Sylvanio Salonensi Interprete)

— Ed. Basileæ, 1537. 8° contains together with another work, a translation of the Definitiones Medicæ (Inscr. Definitiorum medicinalium liber . . . Jona Philologo interprete), *543 a. 2 (1)* [B.M.]. This is an imperfect copy, title page and following leaf is wanting ; another copy is *540 b. 1* [B.M.]

— Claudii Galeni Pergameni definitiones medicæ Jona Philologo interprete. Parisiis, 1528. 8° *540 b. 12 (2)* [B.M.]

— Another edition. Lugduni, 1539. 8° *540 b. 17 (2)* [B.M.]

— See BALLONIUS (G.) G. Ballonii definitionum medicarum liber, in quo . . . sæpe loci . . . Galeni obscuri explicantur &c. 1639. 4° *1167 i. 4 (2)* [B.M.]

— De his quæ pertinent ad definitionem medicinæ propositam a Galeno. See CAMERARIUS (J. R.) Disputationum medicarum . . . decus prima. Disp. I. 1611. 8° *1179 d. 2 (1)* [B.M.]

— See ROESLIN (H.) Disputatio de his quæ pertinent ad definitionem medicinæ propositam a Galeno &c. 1569. 4° *1179 d. 2 (15)* [B.M.]

(110)

ὅτι αἱ ποιότητες ἀσώματοι

Quod qualitates incorporeæ sint

Greek MSS. are known.

Latin translations

— C. V, Isag. f. 25 (Inscr. Claud. Galeno Adscriptus Liber, quod Qualitates incorporeæ sint, Horatio Limano Interprete)

(111)

περὶ χυμῶν

De humoribus

Greek MSS. are known.

Latin translations

— See Hippocrates. ed. 1562. 8° *540 b. 8* [B.M.] which contains " Galeni in Hippocratis librum de humoribus ".

(112)

περὶ προγνώσεως

De prænotione

Greek and Latin MSS. are known. A Latin MS. is Bibl. monast. Gaybac. fol. 285.

Latin translations

— C. II, f. 1567 (Inscr. Claudii Galeni de Prænotione Liber, Jano Cornario Medico Interprete. Argumenta Capitum Quatuordecim Libri Galeni de Præcognitione, ut Leonardi Jachini translationi inserta sunt)

(113)

πρόγνωσις πεπειραμένη καὶ παναληθής

Præsagitio omnino vera expartaque

Greek MSS. are known.

Latin translations

— C. IV, f. 1071 (Inscr. Claudio Galeno Adscriptum præsagium experientia confirmatum. Georgio Valla Placentino interprete)

(114)

περὶ φλεβοτομίας

De venæ sectione

Greek, Arabic, and Latin MSS. are known. A Latin MS. is Parisin. 7416 ; s. xv, (De flebotomia).

Latin translations

— C. III, f. 981 (Josepho Tectrando Craconiemsi Interprete)
Inscr. *Claud. Galeni De Venœ Sectione, Advirsus Erasistratœos,
qui Romœ degebant, Liber.*

(115)

περὶ κατακλίσεως νοσούντων προγνωστικὰ ἐκ τῆς μαθη-
ματικῆς ἐπιστήμης

Prognostica de decubita ex mathematica scientia

Greek MSS. are known. This is said to be a supposititious
work of Galen.

Latin translations

— C. IV, f. 839 (Inscr. Claudio Galeno Adscriptus Liber, cui)
— Prognostica de decubitu . . . liber Galeno ascriptus
J. A. Mariscotto interprete. See VIRDUNG (J.) J. Hasfurti
De cognoscendis et medendis . . . morbis ex corporum clestium.
positione . . . libri IIII. 1584. 4° *788 f. 22* [B.M.]

— Claudii Galeni Pergameni mathematices scientiæ prognostica de decabitu infirmorum, J. Struthio interprete, cum
paraphrasi C. Fabri . . . novissime juncta. Lugduni, 1550. 8°
540 b. 14 (1) [B.M.]

(116)

περὶ οὔρων

De urinis

This is said to be a supposititious work of Galen. Greek,
Arabic, Latin, and Hebrew MSS. are known, and of these a
preponderating number are Greek.

Latin MSS.

Glasgow : Hunterian. T. 4. 13 ; s. x (ix) f. 96 (Liber de
intellectu urinarum ratione nebular. Inc. Inter
omnia quæ de febribus scripta sunt. Expl.
super nebula non periclitatur)

London : Harleian. (Br. Mus.) 4346 ; s. xii, f. 62 (De urinarum
      specie epist. Inc. Primo ostendendum est
      unde urina oritur. Expl. mortifera est)
    Sloan. 1313 ; s. xv, f. 38
        3531 ; s. xv, f. 14–18

Madrid : Matrit. bibl. nac. 1122 (ol. L 195) ; s. xvi, f. 1 (Ex
      Gal. et Hipp. de urinis)

Montecassino : Casinens 97 ; s. x, p. 26 (De pulsibus et urinis.
      Inc. omnium causarum. Explicit initiam
      canculi facit)

Munich : Monac. 505 ; s. xv, f. 122
        11343 (Polling. 43) ; s. xiii, f. 2. [Epist. de
      urinis]

Oxford : Coll. Merton. 219 ; s. xiv in f. 252 (Inc.—talens
      videntes. Explicit dolorum significat. Fort.
      Galeni)

Rome : Barverin. IX 29=767 ; s. —, f. 136

St. Gallen : Sangall. 751 ; s. ix, p. 324–33

Wolfenbüttel : Guerferbyt. 2156 (12. 4. Aug.); s. xv, f. 414–15

Latin translations

— C. II, f. 1249 (Inscr. Claud. Galeni De Urinis, Liber
Spurious, Jano Cornario Medico interprete. Argumenta Capitum
in Librum de Urinis, perperam Galeno adscriptum. Citatur
Galenus cap. 3. Et cap 16, alter de urinis tractatus incipit.
Inter caput 13 & 14, multa leguntur in Græcis superflue, quæ
Cornarius recte omnisit)

De urinis—Greek & Latin

— Liber Galeni de urinis . . . una cum commentariis . . .
Ferdinandi a Mena . . . eodem autore interprete. Greek &
Latin. Compluti. 1553. 4° *540 e. 11 (3)* [B.M.]

— Galeno ascriptus Græcus liber de urinis, ab innumeris
mendis repurgatus et donatus Latinitate studio D. S. Alberti.
Greek & Latin. Vitæbergæ. 1586. 8° *540 b. 17 (3)* [B.M.]

De urinis—Appendix

— See MARTINI (H.) H. Martinii . . . anatomia Urinæ . . .
ex Doctrina Hippocratis and Galeni &c. 1658. 12° *1189 a. 7*
[B.M.]

(117)

πϵρὶ οὔρων ἐν συντόμῳ

De urinis compendium

Greek MSS. are known. Another doubtful Galenic work.

(118)

πϵρὶ οὔρων ἐκ τῶν ῾Ιπποκράτους καὶ Γαληνοῦ καὶ ἄλλων τινῶν

De urinis, ex Hippocrate Galeno aliisque quibusdam

A doubtful Greek MS. survives at Paris. The Latin MS.
Matrit. bibl. nac. 1122 (ol. L 195) ; s. xvi, f. 1 (ex Gal. et Hipp.
de urinis) is of interest if compared to the Greek MS. Parisin.
2269. The matter of the origin of this work still remains to be
cleared up. Works Nos. 116, 117, and 118 pending further
research must in the meantime be classed among the "supposititious works of Galen".

— C. IV, f. 1077 (Georgio Valla Placentino Interprete)
Inscr. *De urinæ significatione ex Hippocrate.* In this tome the
work is placed among the spurious Galenic writings.

(119)

πϵρὶ σφυγμῶν πρὸς ᾿Αντώνιον

De pulsibus ad Antonium

Greek MSS. are known.

(120)

πϵρὶ τῆς τῶν ἐν νϵφροῖς παθῶν διαγνώσϵως καὶ θϵραπϵίας

De affectuum renibus insidentium dignotione et curatione liber

Greek MSS. are known. This is one of the doubtful works.

Latin translations

— Galeni de renum affectus dignotione et medicatione liber ; interprete C. Sotere. Apud J. Schoeffer-Moguntiæ. 1530. 8° *7615 a. 27* [B.M.]

— Claudii Galeni de renum affectus agnitione vel de calculo liber. Parisiis 1535. 8° *540 d. 2 (1)* [B.M.]

— C. III, f. 1535 (Christophoro Heyl Vuisbadensi Interprete)

(121)

περὶ μελαγχολίας ἐκ τῶν Γαληνοῦ καὶ ʻΡούφου καὶ
Ποσειδωνίου καὶ Μαρκέλλου Σικαμίου τοῦ ʼΑετίου βιβλίον

*De melancholia ex Galeno, Rufo, Posidonio et Marcello Sicamii
Ætii libellus*

Greek MSS. are known.

Latin translations

— C. IV, f. 1183 (Jano Cornario medico Interprete)

(122)

περὶ αντεμβαλλομένων

De succedaneis liber

Greek and Latin MSS. are known. One of the supposititious works of Galen.

Latin MSS.

Brussels : Bruxell. 1342–50 ; s. xii, f. 106 (Inc. Pro aloe
mittis licium. Expl. Pro zinzibar mittis piretrum)
Cambridge : Cantabr. Caius Coll. 97 : s. xii–xiii, f. 137b
(Inc. Pro asmanto folia bete [?])
Florence : Laurent.-Leopold (Acd. Flor. Eccl.) 165* ; s. xv,
f. 292
Glasgow : Hunterian. T. 4. 13 ; s. x (ix), f. 15 (Inc. Antiball.
Hipp. et Gal. Inc. Pro acanti sparma. Expl.
pro. zinzibar posatrum=Bruxell.)

Montecassino: Casinens. 69; s. ix, p. 524 (similar to Bruxell.)
Oxford : Bodleian. MSS. Angl. 3637 (Gal. epist. in Anti-
   ballomenon librum)
Paris : Parisin.   6882 ; s. xiii (?)
                   7056 ; s. xiii, f. 121–2
                   11219 ; s. ix, f. 230
                   12999 ; s. xii, f. 2 (Initio mutil.)
Rome :   Regin. 1260 ; s. x, f. 174 (Inc. Pro arganta. Expl.
         pro vilocasia bratans) et f. 178 (Inc. Pro aromatico.
         Expl. silbidio upsala)
     Inscr. *Liber qui intitulater quid pro quo*
     Inc. Quoniam antibellomenon librum et Dioscorides
         noscitur fuiore
     Expl. oleum simplum, ubi sint balanstie
Erfurt : Amplon. F 275 ; s. xiii, xiv, f. 117–8
                  Q 185 ; s. xiii. XIV, f. 6–6 (Epist. Gal.
                     quid pro quo. Inc. In ep. Gal. in
                     Antiballomenon. Expl. pro zinzibar
                     piretrum=Bruxell. above)
Oxford : Coll. B. Mariæ Magd. 164 ; s. xv in f. 43

Latin translations

— De succidaneis. See Blemmidas (N.) G. Valla . . .
interprete . . . Micephoria logica &c. 1498 fol. *8461 f. 6* [B.M.]

(123)
περὶ μέτρων καὶ σταθμῶν
De ponderibus et mensuris

Greek and Latin MSS. are known. A Latin MS. is Laudunens.
418 ; s. xiv/xv, No. 10. This is a supposititious work of Galen.

Latin translations

— C. III, f. 955 (Inscr. Claud. Galeni de Mensuris, ac
Ponderibus, Libellus, Spurious. Jano Cornario Medico Physico
Interprete)

— De Mensuris et Ponderibus, libellus Galeni . . . emendatus.
Greek and Latin. (H. Stephani tractatus de Mensibus et partibus
eorundem.) See Estienne (H.) 2nd of the name. θησαυρὸς
τῆς Ἑλληνικῆς γλώσσης &c. Vol. 12. Part 2. 1816 &c. fol.
1333 1. 5 [B.M.]

— See Pernice (Ericus) Galeni de ponderibus et mensuris
testimonia &c. 1888. 8° *8530 g. 40 (6)* [B.M.]

(124)

περὶ αἰσθήσεων

De quinque sensibus

A single Greek MS. is said to be at Venice (Bibl. Josephi de
Aromatariis), but its whereabouts is not known.

(125)

περὶ αλειμμάτων

De unguentis

A single Greek MS. is known [Jerusalem : Bibl. patriarch.
148 ; s. xvi, f. 40 (π. ἀλ. ἐκ τοῦ Ἱππ. καὶ Γαλ. καὶ ἑτέρων
φιλοσ. κ. ἰατρ.)]

(126)

περὶ ἀνατομῆς

De anatomia

Greek, Arabic and Latin MSS. are known.

Latin MSS.

Bamberg : Bibl. publ. 1691 (L III 37)* ; s. xv (De anatomia
porci)

Basle : Basil. D III 8 ; s. — (De membr. int. seu Anatomia
internar. partium)

Bruges : Bibl. publ. 468 ; s. xiii (Anatomia membrorum
interior)

470 ; s. xiv (Anon. Inc. Calenus in tegni)

Cambrai :   Camaracens. 916 (815) ; s. xiii, f. 106 (Similar to
   Bruges 470)
Cambridge : Cantabr. St. Petri 1862 ; s. —
Douaneschingen : Bibl. Fuerstenberg. 789 ; s. xv (Anatomia
   Ga[leni] plena quam componit Gilbertus)
Douai : nr. 553 ; s. xiv, No. 14 (Similar to Bruges 470)
Erfurt : Amplon. F 289 ; s. xiii, f. 86 (Similar to Bruges 470)
Erlangen : Bibl. Univ. 707 ; a. 1460, f. 246–51
Eton : Bibl. Coll. 132 ; s. xiii, No. 9
Laon : Laudunens. 417 ; s. xiv, No. 4 (Similar to Bruges 470)
Leipzig : Lipsiens. Bibl. Univ. Repos. med. I 4
Leyden : Vossian. 2127 ; s. —
Munich : Monac.   161 ; s. xiii, f. 47
      13034 (Rat. civ. 34) ; s. xiv, f. 48 [Anatomia
        de interioribus]
Oxford : Coll. Merton. 685 ; s. — (De interioribus membris)
Paris : Bibl. de l'Arsenal 865 ; s. xiii, f. 94 (Similar to Bruges
   470)
Rome : Palat. 1144 ; s. —, f. 64 (Similar to Bruges 470)
Turin : Taurin. bibl. reg. G IV 3 (549–K V 31) ; s. xiv, f. 144
   (Similar to Bruges 470)
   Car. Theyer. 6605

Latin translations
— C. IV, f. 949 (Anon. Interprete)

(127)

περὶ τῆς ἀνατομῆς ἐπὶ τῶν ζώντων
De anatomia vivorum

Inc. Medicorum anathomicos necesse est præcognoscere
Expl. diversitas inter Gal. et Aristotelem.
The Greek MSS. have not been identified with any certainty.
Latin MSS.
Cambridge : Cantabr. St. Petri 225 ; s. xiv, f. ix 1 (Expl. mut. :
   ex carne forti et grossa)

Chartres : Autricens. 284 (340) ; s. xiii, f. 139

Munich : Monac. 465 ; a. 1503, f. 110 (Apogr. libri Venetiis
a. 1503 editi)

Oxford : Coll. Balliol. 231 ; s. xiv, in. f. 26

Rome : Palat. 1094 ; s. xiv, f. 212

Vatic. 2383 ; s. —, f. 21

Latin translations

— D. II, f. 294

— C. IV, f. 953 (Anon. Interprete)

(128)

περὶ ἀνέμων, περὶ πυρός, περὶ ὕδατος ὀμβρίου καὶ ὕδατος
ποταμοῦ καὶ ὕδατος θαλασσίου καὶ ὕδατος λίμνης καὶ ὕδατος
φρέατος, ἔτι καὶ τῆς λευκῆς καὶ κοκκινης

De ventis, igne, aquis, terra

Greek MSS. are known.

(129)

περὶ ἀνεντάτων

De non intentis

Known in the Greek manuscript.

(130)

περὶ ἀνθράκων

De carbunculis

A Greek MS. is known.

(131)

περὶ ἀπεψίας

De cruditate

A single Greek MS. is known.

(132)

περὶ ἀποδείξεων

De demonstrationibus

Greek MSS. are known.

(133)

λεξικὸν βοτανικόν

Lexicon botanicum

Greek MSS. are known.

(134)

περὶ γάλακτος

De lacte

Greek MSS. are known. One at Florence (Laurent. ap. Bandini
111 122 De sero lactis) is not Galen's work.

(135)

περὶ γενέσεως

De generatione

This work is known in the Greek manuscripts.

(136)

περὶ γονορροίας

De nimia seminis profusione

A Greek MS. is known.

(137)

περὶ γυναικείων

De gynæceis i.e. de passionibus mulierum

Greek, Latin, and Hebrew MSS. are known.

Latin MSS. (Inc. de passionibus mulierum. Expl. cum vino
cum vino calido libat.)

Dresden : Dresd. Db 92, 93 ; s. xv, f. 256b

Leipzig : Lipsiens. bibl. univ. Repos. med. I 5 ; s. —. (De
sterilitate mulierum. De conceptu mulierum)

Madrid : Matrit. bibl. nac. 4234 (ol. L 163)* ; s. xiii, f. 12
(Inc. Utile prævidi bovis scribere. Expl. f. 21 nec.
lavetur diebus septem)
Paris : Parisin. 6865 ; s. xiv, f. 210d

Latin translations

— D. II, f. 85 (Nicolao de Regio interprete)

— C. IV, f. 1133 (Inscr. Claudio Galeno Adscriptus Liber De
Gynæceis, Id est De Passionibus Mulierum, Nicolao de Regio
Calabro Interprete)

(138)

διαίρεσις

Distinctio

Greek MSS. are known.

(139)

περὶ διαίτης

De victus ratione

Greek MSS. are known.

(140)

περὶ διαίτης καὶ θεραπειῶν πρὸς 'Αντικένσορα Πατρίκιον

De diæta et morbis curandis

Greek MSS. are known.

(141)

εἰσαγωγὴ διαλεκτική

Institutio logica

Known in the Greek manuscript.

(142)

περὶ τῶν ἑαυτῷ δοκούντων

De propriis placitis

Greek and Latin MSS. are known.

Latin MSS.

  Bourges : Biturigens. 299 (247) ; ѕ. xiv, f. 140
  Cesena : Malatest. S V 4 : s. xiv, f. 148–50
  Dresden : Dresd. Db 92, 93 ; s. xv, f. 12b
  Paris : Parisin. 6865 ; s. xiv, f. 172a

Latin translations

  — C. V, Isag. f. 33 (Inscr. Claudii Galeni de Libris propriis
Liber, A. Joanne Fichardo Francofordiano Latinitate Donatus)

(143)

περὶ ἐγκεφάλου καὶ μηνίγγων

De cerebro eiusque tunicis

A single Greek MS. is known.

(144)

περὶ ἐθῶν

De consuetudinibus

Greek and Latin MSS. are known.

Latin MSS.

  Cesena : Malatest. S V 4 ; s. xiv, f. 38
                         S XXVI 4 ; s. xiii, f. 29
  Munich : Monac. 490 ; a. 1488–1503, f. 69, 77
  Oxford : Oxon. Coll. Omn. Animar. 68 ; s. xiv, xv, f. 190
  Paris :   Parisin. 6865 ; s. xiv, f. 73a
  Rome :   Palat. 1098 ; s. xv, f. 2
                    1298 ; s. —, f. 214
            Vatic. 2384 ; s. —, f. 27
                    2417 ; s. —, f. 274

Latin translations

  — D. I, f. 118 (Nicolao de Regio interprete)
  — Regiæ Frederico Alexandrinæ literarum universitatis
prorector . . . successorem suum civibus academicis commendat.
Galeni libellum περὶ ἐθῶν recensuit Iwanus Mueller, p. 19.
Erlangæ, 1879. 4° *773 1. 25* (7) [B.M.]

(145)

περὶ ἐκτρώσεως [?]

De abortivo fœtu

Greek MSS. are known.

(146)

περὶ ἑλκῶν

De vulneribus

Known in Greek manuscript. See Section [261]

(147)

περὶ τῆς ἰατρικῆς ἐμπειρίας

="Sermo adversus empiricos medicos"

Galeni de optimo docendi genere liber, adnotabant et emendabant seminarii philogorum Bonnensis sodales; accedit libri adversus empiricos fragmentum. . . . Gr. cum Lat. Gadaldini versione H. Schœne . . . Bonnæ, 1906.

Greek and Latin MSS. are known. A Latin MS. is *Junt. VII in classe frgm. f. 51.*

Latin translations

— Claudii Galeni de optimo docendi genere liber . . . D. Erasmo interprete. See Sextus, Empiricus. Sexti Empirici . . . adversus Mathematicos . . . opus &c. 1569 fol. *C. 80 e. 4* [B.M.]

De optimo docendi genere—Greek & Latin

— Claudii Galeni Pergameni de optimo docendi genere liber (with the Latin translation of D. Erasmus). See Sextus Empiricus Σέξτου Ἐμπειρικοῖ τὰ σωζόμενα &c. 1621 fol. *722 m. 15* [B.M.]

(148)

πρὸς Γαῦρον περὶ τοῦ πῶς ἐμψυχοῦται τὰ ἔμβρυα

Ad Gaurum quomodo animetur fetus

Known in the Greek manuscript.

(149)

περὶ ἐνυπνίων

De insomniis

Known in the Greek manuscript.

Latin translations

— C. II, f. 1565 (Inscr. Claud. Galeni De Dinotione ex Insomniis Libellus, Jano Cornario Medico Interprete)

(150)

περὶ ᾽Επικτήτου

Galeni et Simplicii testimonia de Epicteto

Known in the Greek manuscript.

(151)

περὶ ἑπταμήνων βρεφῶν

De septimestri partu

Known in the Greek manuscript.

Latin translations

— C. I, f. 1071 (Joanne Bernardo Feliciano Interprete)

— See Hippocrates, ed. 1518 [*C. 79 f. 6 (1)* B.M.]. Nem in libros Hippocratis de Septimestri et . . . partu et . . . in eorum Galeni commentaria, Cardani Commentarii &c. (With the text)

(152)

περὶ ἐρυσιπέλατος

De erysipelate

Known in the Greek manuscript.

(153)

περὶ ζωῆς καὶ θανάτου

De vita et morte

Greek and Latin MSS. are known.

Latin MSS. (See Prognostica de decubitu infirmorum)

(154)

περὶ ζῴων

De animalibus

Greek and Latin MSS. are known. A Latin MS. is at Oxford (Coll. Jesu 99C; s. xvi. Opus de animalium differentiis ex scriptis Arist. Diosc. Plin. Gal. collectum)

(155)

περὶ ζῴων φθαρτικῶν

De animalibus noxiis

Greek MSS. are known.

(156)

περὶ ἥπατος

De iecore

A Greek manuscript is known.

(157)

περὶ θηριακῆς

De theriaca

Greek and Latin MSS. are known.

Latin MSS.

Cesena : Malatest. S. V 4 ; s. xiv, f. 155 (Ad Ceasarum De commoditatibus tyriace. Inc. Quod multa sit apponenda diligentia. Expl. conveniosos esse mihi videtur hoc farmacum)

S. XXVI 4 ; s. xiii, f. 108 (Similar to S V 4)

Dresden : Dresd. Db 92. 93 ; s. xv, f. 192d (De tiriaca et metridato. Inc Medici nominaverunt ea quibus curant. Expl. cum melle rosaceo quod sufficiat)

Florence : Laur.—Leop. (Gadd.) 93 ; s. xiii, f. 118 (Tyriacha Gal. Inc. Trociscorum squilliticorum ÷ XVI. Expl. piperis longi ÷ XII 3 IIII)

Latin translations

— D. II, f. 207 (Nicolao de Regio interprete)

(158)

περὶ θλάσματος

De contusionibus

A Greek MS. is known.

(159)

περὶ ἰατρικῆς τέχνης

De arte medica

Greek, Arabic and Latin MSS. are known. A Latin MS. is at Florence, Riccard. 1165 (L III 34) ; s. xv, f. 96b (Practica et Theorica. Inc. Succinti sermonis eloquio   Expl. quod a nigris concluditur)

(160)

περὶ τῶν ιβ′ θυρῶν [πυλῶν ?]

De XII portis

Greek and Latin MSS. are known.

Latin MSS.

Basle : Basil. D III 8 ; s. — (De XII portis medicinæ microtechn.)

Breslau : Vratisl. bibl. univ. IV F 25 ; s. xiii, f. 199 (De
XII portis)

(161)

ἰατροσοφία

Iatrosophia

Greek MSS. are known.

(162)

περὶ ἰατρῶν

De medicis

Greek and Latin MSS. are known.

Latin MSS.

Rome : Vatic. 2376 ; s. —, f. 209 (Epist. G. de instructione
medici. Inc. Hortor te, o medice, et
hortando moneo. Expl. qui sit
benedictus in sæcula sæculorum.
Amen.)
2417 ; s. —, f. 275 (Similar to 2376)

(163)

ἱππιατροσόφιον

Hippiatrosophium

Greek MSS. are known.

(164)

τοῦ Ἱπποκράτους εἰς τὰ ἀναλυτικὰ βιβλία ιδ', καὶ ἐξηγεῖται
αὐτὰ ὁ Γαληνός

Hippocratis liber resolutionis, quem Galenus explicat

Greek MSS. are known.

(165)

εἰς Ἱπποκράτους περὶ ἡλικιῶν νοσημάτων

In libr. Hippocratis de ætatum ægritudinibus

A Greek manuscript is said to be at Venice.

(166)

περὶ προσοχῆς καὶ προγνώσεως τῶν μελλόντων καθαίρεσθαι

De dignotione hominum purgandorum

A Greek MS. is at the British Museum.

(167)

παραγγελίαι

Scholion in Hippocratis

Known in the Greek manuscript. [Ed. Daremberg : Not. et
Extr. des mscrts. med. I, Paris, 1853, pp. 200–2]

(168)

πῶς χρὴ ἐπιβοηθεῖν τοῖς ποιοῦσι (leg. πιοῦσι) φάρμακον καὶ μὴ καθαιρομένοις

Qua ratione adiuvandi ii sint, qui remedio hausto non purgantur

Known in the Greek manuscript.

(169)

διαθήκη περὶ τῆς τοῦ ἀνθρωπείου σώματος κατασκευῆς. περὶ τῆς τεσσάρων τῶν ὡρῶν τε καὶ ιβ' μηνῶν διαίτης

De hominis natura testamentum. De victu singulis mensibus servando

Known in the Greek MSS.

(170)

περὶ κεφαλαλγίας

De doloris capitis

Known in the Greek MSS.

(171)

περὶ κυνάγχης

De angina

Known in the Greek manuscript.

(172)

περὶ λεπτυνούσης διαίτης

De victu attenuante

Greek and Latin MSS. are known.

Latin MSS.

Cesena : Malatest. S V 4 ; s. xiv, f. 139
             S XXVI 4 ; s. xiii, f. 127
Dresden : Dresd. Db 92, 93 ; s. xv, f. 308d

Paris : Parisin. 6865 ; s. xiv, f. 191b

            14390 ; s. xiv, f. 306 (Sub tit. De diæta acutorum ægritudinum)

Rome : Vatic. 2384 ; s. —, f. 87

Venice : Marcian. 317 ; s. —, p. 137 (Sub tit. De regimine sanitatis)

Latin translations

— D. I, f. 138

— C. I, f. 1206 (Inscr. Claud. Galeni De attenuante victus ratione Liber Unus, Martino Gregorio Interprete)

— Γαληνου περὶ λεπτυνούσης διαίτης. Galeni de victu attenuante liber. Primum Græce edidit Carolus Kalbfleisch Greek. pp. XXV. 44. Leipsiæ. 1898. 8° *2048 g. 4* [B.M.]

— Part of the " Bibliotheca Scriptorum Græcorum et Romanorum Tenbueriana "

(173)

περὶ λέπρας

De lepra alba

Known in the Greek manuscript.

(174)

περὶ λίθων

De lapidibus

A single Greek MS. survives at Madrid. " Hic commentarius apud Iriarte impressus ex Dioscuride Aëtio Galeno aliis consutus est."

Latin translations

— C. IV, f. 1193 (Inscr. Claudio Galeno Adscriptus Liber De Bura Lapidis. Inc. Canon, quem scripsit albuleizor filius Abumelech Filuzer Imperatori Saracenorum—)

(175)

περὶ μετάλλων

De metallis

Known in the Greek manuscript. "Aristotelis et Gal. frgta. de metallis quæ reperiuntur in Cypro insula" (vide Diels: Handschriften d. ant. Ärtze. 1)

(176)

περὶ μηχανημάτων

De machinamentis

Known in the Greek manuscript.

(177)

περὶ σώματος μοριων

De corporis partibus

Known in the Greek manuscript (Frgm. Galeni)

(178)

περὶ νόσων

De morbis excerpta

Greek and Latin MSS. are known.

Latin MSS.

Erfurt : Amplon. Q 343 ; s. xiv, f. 149–56 (Ex Gal. libris, quibus de accidente et morbo et de acutis ægritudinibus inscribitur)

Paris : Parisin. 544 ; s. xiii, No. 1
            7418 ; s. xiv (Exposito de infirmis)

Rome : Palat. 1207 ; s. —, f. 22 (Metrum de morbis. Inc. Morbum describi)

St. Gallen : Sangal. 752 ; s. x–xi, f. 179–326 (Oxæ et chroniæ passiones Hipp. Gal. Sor.)

Inscr. *Passionarius. De passionibus et cura libri III*
Inc. *Cephalea est dolor capitis*

Brussels : Bruxell. 14322/23 ; s. x, f. 1. (Libri VII ut vid.
Expl. f. 89 et molæ fiunt ad triticum frangendum)

Cambridge : Cantabr. Caius Coll. 161 ; s. xii, f. 1b (Expl. lib.
VII : antea quæ sunt futura)

Cheltenham : Philipps. 6956* ; s. — (Gal. [?] de dolore
capitis) sold ?

Dresden : Dresd. Db 92, 93 ; s. xv, f. 509a (Inc. Si quis
intente desiderat. Expl. blando more dintis-
sime perfricando)

Edinburgh : Advocates' Libr. A. 6 41 (18, 6, 13) ; s. xi,
ex.–xii, f. 1 (Libri VII. Expl. perfricando)

Erfurt : Amplon. Q 202 ; s. xii (Libri VII. Expl. similar to
Dresdens)

Escurial : Scorial. N III. 17 ; s. xii, f. 41, 81 (Libri VI. ad
Glaucon. Inc. Quoniam quidem. Expl. serum
curam)

London : Addit. (Br. Mus.) 21, 995 ; s. xii, f. 3
Regius 12 E XX ; s. xii, f. 33 (Gal. philos. ad
Glaucon. nepot. serum. Similar to Scorial
N. III. 17, f. 41. Liber III inc. Cephalea est
dolor)

Milan : Ambros. C 70 Sup ; s. — (Inscr. Opera medica a Gal.
composita et Glauco nepoti suo missa)
D 2 Inf. ; s. — (Libri VII. Expl. in l. VII
c. 39)

Metz : Mediomatric. 509 ; s. xii

Montecassino : Casinens. 97 ; s. x, p. 89 (Des in libro IV.
Expl. commisces et dabis bibere)

Oxford : Coll. Balliol. 231 ; s. xiv in f. 389b (Libri VII.
Expl. plerumque mentes habetantur)

Pisa : Conv. S. Cath. 52 ; s. xii (Libri VII. Expl. similar to
Dresden)

Rome : Urbin. 236 ; s. xiv, f. 91 (Liber Passionarii Gal. de flegmone. Inc. Incipiamus de flegmone dicue. Expl. leves et sorbiles dentur. Explicit chirurgia Passionarii)

Vatic. 4417 ; s. —, f. 37–82 (Libri III de passionibus et cura)

4418 ; s. —, f. 24 (Similar to nr. 4417)

5368 ; s. xiii ? f. 7 (De passionib. et cura libri V. Expl. necesse est loca refrigeratoria facere), et f. 139 (De sinthomatibus. Inc. Nunc diligencius et valde consideremus. Expl. similar to Dresdens)

(179)

ὅρος, τί ἐστι φάρυγξ

Fauces definiuntur

Known in the Greek manuscript.

(180)

περὶ ὀφθαλμῶν

De oculis

Known in the Greek manuscript. It was translated from the Arabic into Latin by Demetrius (see Appendix I. of this work).

Latin translations

— D. I, f. 59 (*De anatomia oculorum*) Inc. Quia oportet secundum amorem. Expl. et amationem boni signavimus)

— C. IV, f. 1001 (Inscr. Claudio Galeno Adscriptus Liber De Anatomia oculorum, Nicolao de Regio Calabro Interprete)

— [See under " De oculis liber adscriptus in VI sectiones distributus "]

(181)

περὶ τῶν παροξυσμῶν χρονων [?]

De paroxysmorum temporibus

Greek MSS. are Parisin. 2269 ; s. xv, f. 151—and 2270 ;
s. xv–xiv, f. 53.

Latin MSS.

    Cesena : Malatest. S V 4 ; s. xiv, f. 34 (Inscr. De tempor.
                parox.)
                S XXVI 4 ; s. xiii, f. 18 (Inscr. similar to
                  S V 4)

    Chartres : Autricens. 293 (351) ; s. xiv, f. 127

    Madrid : Matrit. bibl. nac. 1978 (ol. L 60) ; s. xiv, f. 81

    Paris : Parisin. 6865 ; s. xiv, f. 70b

(182)

περὶ τεττάρων παροξυσμῶν χρόνων

De quattuor temporibus paroxismorum

Known in Greek and Latin MSS.

Latin MSS.

    Cesena : Malatest. S V 4 ; s. xiv, f. 34 (Inscr De temp. parox.)
                S XXVI 4 ; s. xiii, f. 18 (same as above)

    Chartres : Autricens. 293 (351) ; s. xiv, f. 127

    Madrid : Matrit. bibl. nac. 1978 (ol. L. 60) ; s. xiv, f. 81

    Paris : Parisin. 6865 ; s. xiv, f. 70b

Latin translations

  — D. II, f. 38 (Inscr. De quattuor temporibus paroxismorum.
Inc. Qualis animalibus est. Expl. tempora pertransivi solum)

(183)

περὶ ἀρίστης πέψεως τῆς γαστρός

De optima ventris concoctione

Known in the Greek manuscript.

(184)

πρὸς Πατρόφιλον περὶ πλευριτίδος

De laterum morbo ad Patrophilum

Known in the Greek manuscript.

(185)

περὶ τῶν ἐν τῷ Πλάτωνος Τιμαίῳ ἰατρικῶς εἰρημένων

De iis, quæ medice scripta sunt in Platonis Timæo, fragmentum

Known in the Greek manuscript.

Latin translations

— Chartier V p. 275–84. Juntin. VII. Frgm. f. 43. (See Diels : Handschriften d. ant. Ärtze. 1. p. 129)

— C. IV, f. 159 (Inscr. Claudii Galeni in Librum Hippocratis, qui quæ in Medicatrina fiunt, inscribitur, Commentariorum Liber Primus, Joanne Bernardo Feliciano Interprete)

(186)

περὶ ποδάγρας

De podagra

Greek and Latin MSS. are known.

Latin MSS.

Cesena : Malatest. D XXIII, 1 ; s. xiii
Escurial : Scorial. N. III, 17 ; s. xii, f. 130
Rome : Vatic. 4417 ; s.—, f. 82–5 (Inc. Podagricorum causas)
4418 ; s. —, f. 101

(187)

προγνωστικά

Prognostica

Greek and Latin MSS. are known.

Latin MSS.

Cambridge : Cantabr. Caius Coll. 97 ; s. xv, f. 138b (Signa
mortis. sec. Gal.)

957 ; s. — (Signa mortis nec.
Gal.)

Cathedr. Vigorn. 760 (Isagoge Joannitii ad
legendos Gal. libros
prognosticorum)

Einsiedeln : Bibl. monast. 356 ; s. x, f. 65 (Prognost. De morbis.
Inc. Si fuerit capitis dolor. Explicit vim
habent)

Erfurt : Amplon. F 236 ; s. xiv, f. 199 (De signis mortis de
vitæ. Inc. Quisquis prima die. Explicit vel
signa de diebus timendis)

Perudia : Perusin. 1173 (N 124) ; s. xiv, *behind* " Recepta
Hipp ". (Undecim hexam, prognost. de morte)

(188)

περὶ πυρετῶν

De febribus

Greek and Latin MSS. are known.

Latin MSS.

Berlin : Phillipps. 1790. 165 ; s. ix/x, f. 29b (Epist. de febrientibus)

Berne : Bernens. 611 ; s. xiii–ix, f. 82–5 (Epist. de febrientibus
Inc. Multa genera febrium nascuntur Explicit
citando frequenter in ipso loco)

Einsiedeln : Bibl. monast. 304 (4 nr. 74) s. ix (De acutis
febribus et periculosis)

Glasgow : Hunterian. V. 3. 2 ; s. x (ix.), f. — (Inc. Quæ vel
quantæ sint febrium diversitatis. Explicit et
difficilis ad curandum)

Naples : Neapolit. VIII D 34 ; s. xiv (Libri VIII–XI alienius
        opius ; sine auctoris nomine. Inc. In hac
        particula febrium curationem. Explicit febris
        de Intredine humorum . . .

Paris : Parisin. 6837 ; s. xiv (De sphemeris febribus libri
        I–III. IV init.)
        11218 ; s. ix, f. 37 (Explicit contraria contrariis
        medicantur)

Rome : Barberin. IX 29–767 ; s. —, f. 48 (Similar to Parisin.
        6837. Libri V)

      Regin. 1004 ; s. xiii, f. 63 (Epist. de febribus)

      Vatic. 5368 ; s. xiii (?) [Similar to Hunterian V. 3. 2.
        Explicit nutriunt homorem cibis abstin-
        eant]

(189)

περὶ σπέρματος

De spermate

Known in the Greek manuscript. (" De spermate ex Aristotele
et Galeno ")

Latin translations

  — C. IV, f. 925 (Anon. Interprete)

(190)

περὶ στοιχείων

De elementis

Known in the Greek manuscript.

Latin translations

  — C. I, f. 1 (Inscr. Cl. Galeni De elementis secundum Hippocratem . . . libri II . . . Nicolao Leoniceno Interprete)

(191)

περὶ στομαχοῦ

De stomacho

Known in the Greek manuscript.

(192)

περὶ σφυγμῶν

De pulsibus

Known in Greek, Arabic, and Latin MSS. The Arabic MS. (Bodl. 333' ; s. xiv, f. 34–47) is an abridgment of the Greek. The Latin MS. is at Montecassino (Casinens. 97 ; s. x, p. 26. De pulsibus et urinis. Inc. Omnium causarum. Expl. initium cauculi facit).

(193)

περὶ ὑαλίων

De vasis vitreis

Known in the Greek manuscript.

(194)

περὶ ὑδάτων

De aquis

Known in Greek and Latin MSS.

Latin MSS.

Paris : Parisin. 6865 ; s. xiv, f. 198a (De bonitate aquarum. Inc. Optimam aquam aptissimam inc. Explicit in foveis remanebit aquæ malitia)

Rome : Palat. 1098 ; s. xv, f. 114 (Similar to Parisin.)

Latin translations

— D. I, f. 128

— C. IV, f. 1065 (Inscr. Claudio Galeno Attributus Liber De Bonitate Aquæ). Anon. Interprete.

(195)

φάρμακα

Remedia

Greek, Syriac, Arabic, Latin, and Hebrew MSS. are known.

Latin MSS.

Basle : Basil. D III 6 ; s. — (Secretorum remediorum . . .
          libellus)
        D III 8 ; s. —
        D III 14 ; s. — (Antidotarium ord. atph.)

Berlin : Phillipps. 1790. 165 ; s. ix/x, f. 70–7 (Ant. gyra Gal.)
          225 ; s. xi, p. 57, 63 (p. 57 hiera fortissima)

Erfurt : Amplon. F. 236 ; s. xiv (De conferantibus et nociois)
          F. 271 ; s. xiii–xiv, f. 56ᵛ (Doses simplicium
          medicinarum)

Munich : Monac.   5 ; s. xiv, f. 9 (Liber farmacorum)
         490 ; a. 1488–1503 (Lib. farmacor.)
        26626 ; s. xv (Simplicia Gal.)

Oxford : Coll. B. Mariæ Magd. 164 ; s. xiv in. f. 11 (Tabula
        medicin. simplic. Inc. Simplices medicinæ veraces
        ex parte sec. Gal.)

Paris : Bibl. Mazarine 3599 ; s. xiii–xiv, f. 1 (Liber Serapidies
        aggregatus in medicinis simplic. ex dictis Dioscor.
        et Gal. et alior. antiquor.)

      Parisin. 7831 ; s. xv [vide Libri Secretorum ad
        Monteum]

St. Gall. : Sangall. 44 ; s. ix, p. 228, 229, 230

Salamanca : Bibl. Univ. 2–4–6 ; s. xvii, No. 3 (Ald. Garzeran
        interpr. De medicamentis purgantibus)

Wolfenbüttel : Guerferbyt. 1615 (1. 8. Aug.) ; s. xiv, xv,
        f. 116–211 (Similar to Paris. Bibl. Mazarine
        3599)

Latin translations

C. III, f. 1393 (Inscr. Cl. Galeni De remediis paratu facilibus,
libellus, ab Huberto Barlando Philiatrio Latino Sermoni traditus,
& a Junio Paulo Crasso medico Patauino accuratissime castigatus,
& ab omni labe purgatus, addito etiam principio, quod antea
desiderabatur)

— C. III, f. 1421 (Cl. Gal. . . . Liber de medicinis facile parabilibus, ad Solonem Medicorum principem, sine principio. Junio Paulo Crasso Patauino Interprete. Obseruato multa nos in sine istius libri ex veteri translatione apposuisse quæ in Græco codice non vidimus)

— C. III, f. 1455 (Liber Tertius De Medicamentis, quæ ad manum, sunt Faleno adscriptus)

(196)

περὶ ὕλης ἰατρικῆς
De materia medica

Known in the Greek manuscript.

(197)

περὶ εἰδῶν φιλοσοφίας
De partibus philosophiæ

Known in the Greek manuscript.

(198)

περὶ φλεβοτομίας
De venæ sectione

Greek, Hebrew, and Latin MSS. are known.

Latin MSS.

Basle : Basil, D 1 5 : s. —

Cambridge : Cantabr. King's Coll. 21 ; s. xiii–xiv, f. 75

Cesena : Malatest. D XXIII 1 ; s. xiii

        S V 4 ; s. xiv, f. 209

Dresden : Dresd. Db 92, 93 ; s. xv, f. 319c

Madrid : Matrit. bibl. nac. 1978 (ol. L 60) ; s. xiv, f. 97

Munich : Monac. 276 ; s. xiv, f. 75

        640 ; s. xv

        3074 (and 74) ; s. xv, f. 127

Paris : Bibl. de l'Arsenal 1027 ; s. xiv, f. 83 (Inc. Propositum est quidem præsentis negotii breviter tractare)

Rome : Palat. 1093 ; s. xiv, f. 126 (Inc. Flebotomia est recta
venæ incisis)
1094 ; s. xiv, f. 487 (similar to 1093)
1098 ; s. xv, f. 79
1111 ; s. —, f. 80
Urbin. 236 ; s.xiv, f. 31 (Inc. Similar to Palat. 1093.
Explicit longioris vitæ saintatem
ministrat)
Vatic. 2376 ; s. —, f. 90
2378 ; s. —, f. 244
2381 ; s. —, f. 200
2385 ; s. —, f. 162
Volterra : Volaterran. 103 (6365) ; s. xv, f. 64
Latin translations
— D. I, f. 145
— C. I, f. 161 (Cl. Gal. De vennarum arteriarumque dissectione Liber, Ab Antonio Fortolo Joseriensi Latinitate donatus,
& ab Andrea Vesalio Bruxellensi plerisque in locis recognitus)

(199)
περὶ φύσεως ἀνβρώπου
De hominis natura

Greek and Latin MSS. are known.
Latin MSS.
Cantabr. Caius Coll. 956 ; s. — (Ep. de humano corpore)
Oxford : Cathedr. Vigorn. 760 ; s. — (De corporis, causis
signis sanis ægris neutris)
Latin translations
— C. I, f. 77 (contains Galen's commentary on Hippocrates'.
De natura humana . . . Herman Cruserio Campensi interprete)

(200)
περὶ χειρουργησιῶν καὶ περὶ κατακλίσεως νοσούντων
De chirurgorum operationibus et de decubitu infirmorum
Known in the Greek manuscript.

(201)

περὶ χειρουργίας

De chirurgia

Greek, Latin and Hebrew MSS. are known. Of these the Hebrew MS. *Monac. 291* (litteris hebr., lingua Hisp.) is of interest as it indicates the position occupied by the Jews in the translating movement in Spain during the Middle Ages.

Latin MSS.

Basle : Basil. D I 12 ; s. (Chirurgia)

Rome : Vatic. 2369 ; s. —, f. 81 (Chirurgia vulnerum liber III et IV)

(202)

περὶ χυμῶν

De humoribus

Known in Greek and Latin MSS.

Latin MSS.

Angers : Andecavens. 461 (446) ; s. xvi, f. 162 (Passarti tract. de humoribus ex Gal. et Hipp. doctrina)

Escurial : Scorial. N. III, 17 : s. xii, f. 99 (Inc. Omnibus hominibus generantur ægritudines ex quatt. humoribus. Expl. sicut in omnibus vulneribus ratio exigit)

Paris : Parisin. 11219 ; s. ix, f. 103 (Epist. Hipp. et Gal. contemplantis quatt. esse humorus in corpore humano. Explicit cum taciturnitate et tristitia alimantur)

Rome : Regin. 1004 ; s. xiii, f. 53 (Similar to Parisinus. Inc. Cephalea est dolor capitis=Gal. Passionarii Inc. Vide under π. νόσων)

(203)

περὶ ὡρῶν καὶ ἔτους

De anni temporibus

Known in the Greek manuscript.

(204)

De accidenti et morbo libri VI

[Probably a translation of π. αἰτίωη συμπτωμάτωη]
Inc. In initio huius libri morbum.
Expl. accidentia semper alia sequuntur quæve non.

Latin MSS.

Angers : Andecavens. 461 (446) ; s. xvi, f. 20 (Jo. Riolani
        annott. in libros VI, ac morborum et symptomatum
        differentiis et causis)

Basle : Basil. D III 8 ; s. — (Inscr. De morborum differentiis
        et causis et De accidentibus seu symptomatibus)

Boulogne-sur-Mer : Bononiens. 197 ; s. xiii, No. 2

Breslau : Vratisl. bibl. univ. IV F 25* ; s. xiii, f. 127–9
                    IV F 26 ; s. —, f. 47–65

Cambrai : Camaracens. 907 (806) ; s. xiv, f. 88

Cambridge : Cantabr. Caius Coll. 98 ; s. xv, f. 81
        St. Petri 33 ; s. xiii/xiv, f. 24

Cesena : Malatest. D XXV 1 ; s. xiii, f. 170
           D XXV 2 ; s. xiii
           S   V 4 ; s. xiv, f. 11

Chartres : Autricens. 284 (340) ; s. xiii, f. 149
              293 (351) ; s. xiv, f. 1 (Inscr. De
              morborum acutorum regimine)

Erfurt : Amplon. F 249 ; s. xiii, f. 90
          F 278 ; s. xiv in. f. 55 (Inc. Primo quidem
             dicere oportet)
          F 280 ; s. xiv, in. f. 114
          F 291 ; s. xiii ex. f. 67
          Q 198 ; s. xiv in. f. 1
          Q 343* ; s. xiv, f. 149

Eton : Bibl. Coll. 132 ; s. xiii, No. 3

Florence : Laurent.-Leopold. (Gaddian.) 58 ; s. xiv, f. 120

Leipzig : Lipsiens. bibl. univ. Repos. med. I 4 ; s. — (De
        accidentibus morborum et causis eorundum)

London : Harleian. (Br. Mus.) 3748 ; s. xv, f. 113
Madrid : Matrit. bibl. nac. 1198 (ol. L 9) ; s. xiv, f. 1. (Inscr.
           Similar to Andecavens. 461)
        1978 (ol. L 60) ; s. xiv, f. 119, 121,
           124, 127, 134. ss. 75–80.
          (Inscr. similar to Andecavens)
        2308 (ol. L 94) ; s. xv, f. 55, 67, 78,
           91, 111, 132
Montecassino : Casinens. 70 ; s. xiv, p. 1
Montpellier : Montepess. (École de méd.) 18 ; s. xiii
Munich : Monac. 5 ; s. xiv, f. 21
      11 ; s. xiv, f. 1
      35 ; s. xiii, xiv, f. 145
Naples : Neapolit. VIII D 30 ; s. xiv
       VIII D 34 ; s. xiv
Oxford : Coll. Balliol. 231 ; s. xiv in. f. 135b
   Coll. Merton. 218 ; s. xiv, f. 77b
       219 ; s. xiv, in. f. 92
Paris : Bibl. de l'Arsenal 1080* ; s. xiv, f. 1 (abbreviat. a
   Joh. de St. Amando)
  Parisin. 6865A ; s. xiv
      9331 ; s. xv
      11860 ; s. xiv, f. 61
      11862 ; s. xvi (De accidentibus)
      14389 ; s. xiv, f. 80
      15455 ; s. xiii, f. 1
      16175 ; s. xiii, f. 63
     Nouv. acq. 1482 ; s. —, f. 36
Rome : Palat. 1092 ; s. —, f. 74
      1093 ; s. xiv, f. 32
      1094 ; s. xiv, f. 229
      1095 ; s. xiv, f. 85
      1096 ; s. xiv, f. 134
      1104 ; s. —, f. 72

Urbin.   235 ; s. xiv, f. 83

247 ; s. xiv, f. 302

Vatic.   2375 ; s. xiv

2378 ; s. —, f. 173

2381 ; s. —, f. 95

2389 ; s. —, f. 81

4451 ; s. xiv, f. 115

Vendôme : Vindocin. 234 ; s. xiv, f. 1

Volterra : Volaterran. 103 (6365) ; s. xv, f. 104

Latin translations

— D. II, f. 2

(205)

De anatomia parva

Inc.   Quoniam interiorum membrorum

Expl. dicitur posticus nervus.

Latin MSS.

London : Sloan. (Br. Mus.) 3566 ; s. xv, f. 127

Munich : Monacens. 465 ; a. 1503 f. 106 (Apogr. libri a. 1503 Venetiis editi)

Rome : Vatic. 2378 ; s. —, f. 62 (Inscr. De anatomia simiæ. Inc. albus et augustus dicitur octiquis)

Würzburg : Wirceburg. med. 4° 1 ; s. xiii, xiv, No. 4

Latin translations

— D. II, f. 294

— C. IV, f. 949 (Caput. I. De anatomia porci 2. De anatomia matricis   3. De anatomia cerebri). This is described as a spurious Galenic work, see f. 3 and 4 of this tome.

(206)

De iuvamento anhelitus

Inc.   Calorem vitalem qui est in corde

Expl. solus veritatis ostensor.

Latin MSS.

Bourges : Biturigens. 299 (247) ; s. xiv, f. 147

Breslau : Vratisl. bibl. univ. IV F 25 ; s. xiii, f. 54 (Cf.
Schneider's Ind. lect. univ. Vratisl. 1840/41)

Cesena : Malatest. D XXV 2 ; s. xiii
S V 4 ; s. xiv, f. 9
S XXVI 4 ; s. xiii, f. 10

Dresden : Dresd. Db 92, 93 ; s. xv, f. 24d

Erfurt : Amplon. F 280 ; s. xiv in. f. 56

Madrid : Matrit. bibl. nac. 1978 (ol. L. 60) ; s. xiv, f. 131

Moulins : nr. 30 ; s. xiv, f. 92

Paris : Parisin. 6865 ; s. xiv, f. 118d
7047 ; s. xiv, No. 2
11860 ; s. xiv, f. 217
15456 ; s. xiii, f. 147

Rome : Palat. 1094 ; s. xiv, f. 568 (Sine tit.)
1097 ; s. —, f. 114

Vatic. 2378 ; s. —, f. 103

Subiaco : nr. 59 ; s. xiii, f. 60

Latin translations

— D. I, f. 84

(207)

De partibus artis medicæ

Inc. De partibus medicativæ, Juste dilectissime, **convenientur**
Expl. et deinde alia secundum prius dictam methodum **adicere.**

Latin translations

— Chart. II, p. 282
— Junt. VII in classe spurior. f. 16
— C. IV, f. 853 (Inscr. Cl. Galeni De partibus artis **medicativæ**
Ad Justum, Nicolao Calabro Interprete)

(208)

Astrologica

Latin MSS.

Avignon : Avennicus 1022 (Auc. fonds 341) ; s. xv, f. 12
(Tract. astrolog. sec. Gal. et Hipp. Inc. Et
quoniam principalis intentio. Explicit si non,
morcitur)

London : Egerton (Br. Mus.) 2433 ; s. xv, f. 47 (Complexiones
hominis astronomiæ et philosophical sec. Gal.)

Munich : Monacens. 276 ; s. xiv, f. 82

(209)

Libre cathagenarum

Latin MSS.

Dresden : Dresd. Db 92, 93 ; s. xv, f. 181c (Inc. Ego quidem
ponam inventionem. Expl. celeriter auferre
prædicta nocumenta)

Paris : Parisin. 6865 ; s. xiv, f. 139b (similar to Dresdens)

Rome : Palat. 1310 ; s. —, f. 73 (Gal. Cathagines. Inc. . . .
iam rettuli)

(210)

De catharticis

Inc. Quoniam cognovimus qualiter Hippocrates
Expl. colligere potiu, habeas experta.

A Latin MS. is Lipsiens, bibl. univ. Repos. med. I. 4 ; s. —

Latin translations

— D. I, f. 149

— C. IV, f. 1127 (Inscr. Cl. Gal. Adscriptus Liber De
Catharticis). Anon. Intpr.

(211)

De virtute centaureæ

Inc. Ego vidi, frater mi Papia
Expl. in tantum dicta sufficiant.

Latin MSS.

Cesena : Malatest. S V 4 ; s. xiv, f. 157

           S XXVI 4 ; s. xiii, f. 124

Escurial : Scorial. f. III, 6 ; s. xv, f. 192

Oxford : Coll. Omn. Animar. 75 ; s. xv, f. 39b (Inc. Ego vidi
      sicut)

Rome : Vatic. 2378 ; s. —, f. 227

           2388 ; s. —, f. 87

Latin translations

— C. IV, f. 1121 (Inc. Ego vidi, frater mi Papia. Expl. in
tantum dicta sufficiant). Nicolao Regio interpr.

— Incipit liber Galeni ad Papia. de virtute cetauree. [Translated by Nicholas Rheginus.] See YUHANNA IBN SERAPION.
Liber Serapionis aggregatus in medicinis simplibicus Vol. I.
1479 fol. *I. B. 20649–50* [B.M.]

— Incipit liber Galeni ad Papia de vtute cetauree. See
YUHANNA IBN SERAPION. Practica Jo. Serapionis dicta
breviarium &c. 1497 fol. *I. B. 22971* [B.M.]

— Liber ad Papiam de virtute centauree. See YUHANNA IBN
SERAPION. Practica &c. 1525 fol. *543 f. 5* [B.M.]

— Incerti autoris de Centaures libellus hactenus Galeno
inscriptus. See YUHANNA IBN SERAPION. In hoc volumine
continentur. Inorginium medicorum &c. 1531 fol. *547 k. 4*
[B.M.]

(212)

De clysteribus et colica

Inc. Conveniens et necessarium est homini volenti audire
medicinam.

Expl. secure et utiliter subveniri.

Hebrew and Latin MSS. are known.

Latin MSS.

Dresden : Dresd. Db 92, 93 ; s. xv, f. 392c (Expl. benedictus
      in sæcula sæculorum)

Paris : Parisin. 6865 ; s. xiv, f. 175b (Expl. similar to Dresd.)

6867 ; s. xv

Latin translations

— Claudii Galeni . . . de clysteribus et colica liber. (Translated into Latin by F. Raphelengius.) Lugduni Bataborum 1591. 8° *540 b. 17 (1)* [B.M.]

(213)

De colera nigra

Inc. De nigra quippe colera

Expl. Hippocratis intentionen sophistizant.

Hebrew and Latin MSS. are known.

Latin MSS.

Cesena : Malatest. S V 4 ; s. xiv, f. 145

S XXVI 4 ; s. xiii, f. 101

Latin translations

— D. I, f. 57 (Petro Dubanensi interpr.)

(214)

De colico dolore libellus

(*See under " De clysteribus et colica "*)

Latin MSS.

Paris : Parisin. 6865 ; s. xiv

6867 ; s. xv

(215)

De causis contentivis

Inc. Stoycos philosophos novi

Expl. auxilia quibus easdestruit assumit.

Latin MSS.

Dresden : Dresd. Db 92, 93 ; s. xv, f. 443a

Paris : Parisin. 6865 ; s. xiv, f. 5

Latin translations
— Ed. Kalbfleisch, Marpurgi Chatt. 1904

(216)

De natura et ordine cuiuslibet corporis
Inc. Licet te sciam, carissime nepos
Expl. suisque temporibus esse curanda.

Latin MSS.
Cambridge : Cantabr: Caius. Coll. 97 ; s. xv, f. 137 (Inscr.
Epist. Gal. de humano corpore. Inc. Licet
te fili carissime. Expl. purgantoriis purganda
sunt)
Munich : Monac. 465 ; a. 1503, f. 175 (Apogr. libri a. 1503
Venetiis editi)

Latin translations
— D. II, f. 302
— C. IV, f. 945 (Anon. Interpr.)

(217)

Diagnostica
Arabic and Latin MSS. are known. The Arabic MS. at Paris is
a fragment. The Latin MS. is Cantabr. St. Joh. D 3 ; s. xiii,
f. 64b (Diagnosticon liber. Inc. Rationem quidem puto. Expl.
mutil. septentrionales quam)

(218)

Dinamidiis
Inc. Verum hæc est virtutis demonstratio
Expl. nulla cura iam superari poterit.

Latin MSS.
Paris : Parisin. 7028 ; s. xi, f. 136 (fine mutil.)
Rome : Regin. 1004 ; s. xiii, f. 42

Latin translations

— D. II, f. 85
— C. IV, f. 861 (Anon. Interpr.)

(219)

Liber alter de Dinamidiis, ad Mæcenatem

Inc. Libellum quem roganti tibi promisi
Expl. mitte flores sipie.

Latin MSS.

Cambridge : Cantabr. Caius Coll. 379 ;   s.   xii/xiii,   f. 55
(Expl. componere velut
creationem)
966 ; s. —
976 ; s. —
St. Petri 33 ; s. xiii/xiv, f. 192 (ad Mæcenatem
de regenda sanitate)
Dresden : Dresd. Db 92. 93 ; s. xv, f. 270c (Expl. inde in
vulvam E. 11)
München : Monac. 465 ; a. 1503, f. 182 (Apogr. libri Venetiis
a. 1503 editi)
Paris : Parisin.   7028 ; s. xi, f. 144 (?)
15113 ; s. xiii, f. 12 (Liber dinam., quem facit
Mæcenati simplicium medicaminum)
15456 ; s. xiii, f. 163
16944 ; s. xii, f. 73
Rome : Palat.   1094 ; s. xiv, f. 606
Vatic.   2378 ; s. —, f. 227
4437 ; s. —, f. 6

Latin translations

— D. II, f. 303
— C. IV, f. 863 (Expl. & Sine dubio liberabitur)

(220)

De dinamidiis
(Varia)

Latin MSS.

Breslau : Vratisl. bibl. acad. Ac. III F 29 ; s. xva, f. 112–28.
(Practica [dinamid.] Gal. scripta in studio
Montepessulani a. 1411)

Cambridge : Cantabr. Caius. Coll. 411 ; s. xiii, f. 169 (De
Inamidiorum [sic] Gal. Inc. Quia disputatio
custodiendæ sanitatis. Des imperf. f. 207b)

London : Addit. (Br. Mus.) 34, III ; s. xv, f. 114 (Experimenta
dinamid. libri Gal.)

Venice : Bibl. monast. St. Michælis (whereabouts not known)

(221)

Dioxe

Greek MSS. are known.

Latin MSS.

Erfurt : Amplon. O 28 ; s. xiii, xiv, f. 45. Inc. Nemo alieno
peccato puisitur. Expl. quod te fecisse pæniteat

Rome : Vatic. 3087 ; s. —, f. 56 (Inc. and Expl. same as in
the preceding)

(222)

De facultatibus corpus nostrum dispensantibus

Inc. De dispensantibus corpus nostrum virtutibus
Expl. intemperantiam et colupattem operat.

Latin MSS.

Basle : Basil. D I 5 ; s. —

Cesena : Malatest. S V 4 ; s. xiv, f. 27
S XXVI 4 ; s. xiii, f. 15

Chartres : Autricens. 293 (351) ; s. xiv, f. 125

Munich : Monacens. 490 ; a. 1488–1503
Paris : Parisin. 6865 ; s. xiv, f. 78d
      7015 ; s. xiv
      Nouv. acq. 343 ; s. xiii, f. 49
Rome : Palat. 1096 ; s. xiv, f. 183
      1096 ; s. xiv, f. 10 et 24
Latin translations
— D. I, f. 102

(223)

De dissolutione contunia s. de alimentorum facultatibus
Latin translations
— Chart. VI, p. 403
— Junt. VII int. spur. f. 71
— C. IV, f. 1051 (Inscr. Cl. Galeno Attributus De dissolutione Continua Corporis Humani, & de natura alimentorum, quibus quod effluxerit restituitur). Anon. Interpr.
— C. I, f. 1082 (Libri III, Martino Gregorio Interprete. Inc. [lib. 1] : De facultatibus, quæ alimentis insunt. Expl. [lib. 3] ; in quibus iandiu habitant, differentias)

(224)

Dogmatice pros haucona (Glaucona ?)
Latin MSS.
Parisin. 12958 ; s. ix (Gal. dogmatice pros haucona lib. primus. Inc. Dum esse difficilis ratio. Expl. saltu suo arteria ambitum)

(225)

De elixir solis et lunæ
Latin MSS.
Jena : Jenens. bibl. acad. 117 ; s. —
Rome : Palat. 1328 ; s. —, f. 41 (Liber secretus super elixir solis et lunæ. Inc. Arbor quæ)

(226)

Epistulæ variæ

Latin MSS.

London : Addit. (Br. Mus.) 8928 ; s. xi, f. 13 (Epist. ad
Titum. Inc. Ne ignorans quispiam
medicorum rationem organi). (See
Hipp. epist.— Casinens. 97, p. 24, No. 3)

Sloan. 1610 ; s. xiv, f. 42 (De regimine sanitatis
pro rege Alexandro conscriptum. Inc.
Cum sit ho corrupt. Expl. usque ad
medium Martis hiems habetur)

Montecassino : Casinens. 225 ; s. xi, p. 34 (Epist. ad Glauconem. Inc. Maximum est medicina ut
primum cognoscas causam. Expl. et
diligenter considerare)

Rome : Regin. 1004 ; s. xiii, f. 42 (Inc. Flegotomarum genera
tria. Cephalargia)

(227)

De usu farmacorum

Inc. De farmicis autem causæ non ut existimatur sunt
Expl. sed clisteri uti, idem enim periculum.

Latin MSS.

Dresden : Dresd. Db 92, 93 ; s. v, f. 392b
Erfurt : Amplon. F 278 ; s. xiv, in. f. 213
Madrid : Matrit. bibl. nac. 1978 (ol. L. 60) ; s. xiv, f. 101
Paris : Parisin. 6865 ; s. xv, f. 179b

(228)

In Hippocratem de aëre, aquis et locis commentarii III

Inc. (lib. 1) : Quicumque artem medicam integre assequi
Expl. (lib. 3) : cæteris nationibus exceptis Ægyptiis cognita
non fuit.

Latin and Hebrew translations are known.

Latin translations
— Chart. VI, p. 187
— Junt. IX, class. 2, f. 1
— C. I, f. 1075 (Inscr. Hippocratis De Æure, Aquis, & Locis, Libellus, Jano Cornario Interprete. Galeni Commentaria desiderantur. Inc. Quicumque artem medicam integre adsequi)

(229)

Quæsita in Hippocratem de urinis

Latin translations
— Chart. VIII, p. 918
— Junt. VII. int. spur. f. 113
— C. IV, f. 1199 (Anon. Interpr.)
— Galeni Quæstiones in Hippocratem. See Valla (G.) G. Vallæ . . . de urinæ significatione &c. 1528. 8° *957 k. 28 (2)* [B.M.]
— 1530 ? 8° *714 a. 15 (1)* [B.M.]

(230)

De cura icteri

Inc. Ad icteri curam
Expl. et hoc est cura ictericorum.

Arabic and Latin MSS. are known.

Latin MSS.
Basle : Basil. D I 5 ; s. —
Cesena : Malatest. S V 4 ; s. xiv, f. 40
S XXVI 4 ; s. xiii, f. 72
Chartres : Autricens. 293 (351) ; s. xiv, f. 124
Dresden : Dresd. Db 92, 93 ; s. xv, f. 465c
Madrid : Matrit. bibl. nac. 1978 (ol. L. 60) ; s. xiv, f. 95
Munich : Monac. 490 ; a. 1488–1503

Paris : Parisin. 6865 ; s. xiv, f. 80b
Rome : Palat. 1098 ; s. xv, f. 8
      Vatic. 2376 ; s. —, f. 211

Latin translations
— D. II, f. 57
— C. IV, f. 1189 (Inscr. Claudio Galeno Attributus Liber De Cura Icteri) Anon. Interpr.

(231)

De incantatione, adjuratione et suspensione
    Inc. Quæsisti, fili carissime, de incantatione
    Expl. magnum sui altitudinem.
Latin MSS.
    Munich : Monac. 465 ; a. 1503, f. 263 (Apogr. libri Venetiis
        a. 1503 editi)
    Rome : Vatic. 2378 ; s. —, f. 61
Latin translations
— D. II, f. 314
— C. III, f. 1497 (Inscr. Cl. Galeno Adscriptus Liber de Incantatione, Adjuratione, & Suspensione. Est autem inter Constantini Africani opera excusus . . . Libri de incantatione, & amuletis, quem inter Constantanti Africani opera legimus)

(232)

De cura lapidis
    Inc. Canon. quem scripsit Alguazir Albuleizor
    Expl. ad pondus drach. II ieiuno stomacho
Latin translations
— Chart. X, p. 546
— Junt. VII int. spur. f. 111
— C. IV, f. 1193 (Anon. Interpr.) Inc. Canon, quem scripsit Alguazir Albuleizor filius abumelech Filuzer Imperatori Saracen-

orum Auley filis Joseph filii Resaptun de curatione lapidis.
Expl. ad pondus drachmarum duarum ieiuno stomacho.

(233)

De medicamentis expertis
Inc. Ignis qui de cælo descendit
Expl. in fine huius tractatus.
Arabic and Latin MSS. are known.

Latin MSS.

Avignon : Avennic. 1019 (Auc. fonds 345) ; s. xiii ex. f. 161
Breslau : Vratisl. bibl. acad. Ac. III F 2* ; s. xv, f. 266–8
Dresden : Dresd. Db 92, 93 ; s. xv, f. 257d
Erfurt : Amplon. F 260 ; s. xiii–xiv, f. 355
Leipzig : Lipsiens. bibl. univ. Repos. med. I 4 ; s. — (Liber
        experimentorum)
Munich : Monacens.   372 ; s. xv, f. 185 (Ferrano interpr.)
                666* ; s. xv, f. 288
                13026 (Rat. civ. 26) ; s. xiv, f. 1 (Inscr.
                   liber de secretis Gal.)
                19901 (Teg. 1901) ; s. xv, f. 209.
                   (Fraartachio interpr.)
Oxford : Coll. Balliol. 285 ; s. xiii, f. 198 (Expl. statim.
        accendatur.)
Paris : Parisin. 6893 ; s. xiv, No. 4
Pavia : Bibl. univ. 10 ; s. xvi, f. 168 (Liber experimentorum)
Rome : Vatic. 2385 ; s. —, f. 266 (Sine titulo trad.)
            2416 ; s. —, f. 24
            2418 ; s. —, f. 84
            4437 ; s. —, f. 16 (Lib. experimentorum)

Latin translations
— D. II, f. 202
— C. IV, f. 1163 (Inscr. Claudio Galeno Attributus Liber De
Medicinis expertis, cui titulus est, Medicinalis experimentatio)
Anon. Interpr.

(234)

De duplici medicina

A Latin MS. is at Turin (Taurinens. ap. Montfaucon. p. 1397).
Latin translations

— C. III, f. 297 (Inscr. Claudii Galeni Liber De Substitutis
Medicinis. Juliano Martiano Rota Inteprete). Inc. De substitutis medicinis cum & Dioscoridem & Philistionem & Eury-
phontem scripsisse constet, nos quod ; pauca de tradere no
recusabimus. Expl. Zingibere—Pyrethrum). This is an interest-
ing work, and the following are typical examples of duplicates or
substitutes. Succo papaveris—Mandragoræ fructus, Refina
pini—Terebinthi, Hyænæ adipe—Vulpis adeps, and Pipere albo
—Nigri duplum. It contains some 350 remedies and their
duplicates, among which are a number indicating Eastern
origin, e.g. Nardus indica, Lotus herba, and Ricini oleum.

(235)

De simplicibus medicinis ad Paternianum

Inc. Cum mihi proposuissem, clarissime Paterniane
Expl. membrum sine ratione mutat.

Latin MSS.
Cues : Bibl. Nic. Cusani. med. 8 ; s. xiii, xiv, No. 5 (De simplic.
medicinis libri V)
Leipzig : Lipsiens. bibl. univ. Repos. med. I 4 ; s. —
I 22 ; s. —
Lucca : Lucens. 296 (B 196) ; s. viii–ix, f. 81
Montecassino : Casinens. 97* ; s. x
Paris : Parisin. 9331 ; s. xv (De simplic. medicinis)
14389 ; s. xiv, f. 280 (De simpl. medicinis)
Rome : Palat. 1094; s. xiv, f. 488 (De simplicibus pharmaciis)
et f. 549 (Inc. Post. quam cœpi
narrare)

Vatic. 2378 ; s. —, f. 145 (Inscr. similar to Cusan.
med. 8 ; libri V)

St. Gall : Sangall. 762 ; s. ix
Vienna : Vindob. 2425 ; s. xi

Latin translations

— D. I, f. 216
— C. IV, f. 1079 (Anon. Interpr.).   Cap. CCL. which is on
Ginger contains the following :—" Iuuentur maxime in Troglo-
dytis, et Arabiæ partibus."   Cap. CCLX contains the following :—" Syrum nascitur in Africa, et in India optimum tame
habetur Arabum, . . ."   Cap. CCLXXVII. reads " Thus,
lacryma est arboris, quæ in Arabia, et in India nascitur, quæ
Græce . . . dicitur.   Quod ergo de Arabiæ arbore manat,
candidius est ; quod de India . . . Expl. in nullo possit reprobus
inueniri.

(236)

De compage membrorum s. de natura humana
Inc. Cerebrum natura quidem frigidum
Expl. membrum sine ratione mutat.

Latin MSS.

Cambridge : Cantabr. Coll. Caii 95 ; s. xiii, f. 10
Munich : Monac. 238 ; s. xv, f. 284

465 ; a. 1503, f. 97 (Apogr. libri Venetiis
a. 1503 editi)

Oxford : Coll. Merton. 278 ; s. xiv, f. 180b (Sine auctoris
nomine)

Latin translations

— D. II, f. 292
— C. IV, f. 1005 (Inscr. Cl. Gal. Adscriptus Liber de Compagine Membrorum, sive de Natura humana. Inc. Cerebrum
natura quidem frigidum. Expl. membrum sine ratione mutat)
Anon. Interpr.

(237)

De minutionibus

A Latin MS. is Monacens. 18444 (Teg. 444) ; s. xv, f. 197

(238)

De morborum et symptomatum differentiis et causis libri VI
(See under " De accidenti et morbi ")

(239)

De morsu, qui in ægritudine percipitur

Latin translations
— Junt. VII. int. spur. f. 63

(240)

De motu thoracis et pulmonis

Inc. Quoniam quidem thorax et pulmonis
Expl. pulmoni princeps motus.

Latin MSS.
Dresden : Dresd. Db 92, 93 ; s. xv, f. 19d
Madrid : Matrit. bibl. nac. 1978 (ol. L. 60) ; s. xiv, f. 131
Paris : Parisin. 6865 ; s. xiv, f. 198a
Rome : Palat. 1098 ; s. xv, f. 10 (Inscr. De dispensantibus
corpus virtutibus. Inc. Quoniam
quidem de thorax (!) movere)
Vatic. 2378 ; s. —, f. 120
2384 ; s. —, f. 67

Latin translations
— D. I, f. 82
— C. I, f. 991 (Anon. Interpr.)

(241)

De motibus liquidis seu De motibus manifestis et obscuris
    Inc. Illi quorum proprium est anatomiam meditari
    Expl. appetitus valde intenditur et superat.

Latin MSS.

Bourges : Biturigens. 299 (247) ; s. xiv, f. 45
Breslau : Vratisl. bibl. univ. IV F 25 ; s. xiii, f. 91–4
Cesena : Malatest. D XXIII 1 ; s. xiii
              D XXV 2 ; s. xiii
              S V 4 ; s. xiv, f. 5
Chartres : Autricens. 284 (340) ; s. xiii, f. 135
Dresden : Dresd. Db 92, 93 ; s. xv, f. 503d (Inscr. De motibus
              liquidis et difficilibus)
Erfurt : Amplon. F 249 ; s. xiii, f. 189
              F 280 ; s. xiv in. f. 42
Montpellier : Montepess. (École de méd.) 18 ; s. xiii
Oxford : Coll. Balliol. 231 ; s. xiv in. f. 51
Paris : Parisin. 6865 ; s. xiv, f. 148b
              11860 ; s. xiv, f. 219
              15456 ; s. xiii, f. 142
Rome : Palat. 1094 ; s. xiv, f. 205
              1099 ; s. xv, f. 67
          Urbin. 247 ; s. xiv, f. 169
          Vatic. 2375 ; s. xiv, f. 472
              2378 ; s. —, f. 222
              2382 ; s. —, f. 56
              2383 ; s. —, f. 37
              2384 ; s. —, f. 42
Volterra : Volaterran. 103 (6365) ; s. xv, f. 131

Latin translations

— D. I, f. 78 (Marco Toletano interpr.)
— C. IV, f. 1033 (Inscr. Cl. Galeno Adscriptus Liber De
Motibus Manifestis et Obscuris, quem Joannitius de Græca

Lingua in Arabicam transtulit, M. autem Toletanus de Arabica in Latinam. Inc. Inquit Galenus, illi, quoru proprium est anatomiam meditari. Expl. appetitus valde intenditur, & superat)

(242)

De oculis liber adscriptus in VI sectiones distributus

(See Hirschberg : Gesch. der Augenheilkunde im Altertum, s. 353 ff., and also section 180 of this volume.)

Latin translations

— Chart. X, p. 504–22
— Junt. VII, cl. VII, f. 182
— C. III, f. 1501 (Inscr. Claud. Galeni de Oculis, a Demetrio translatus, nuper autem a variis mendis expurgatus. Argumenta libri de oculis, cuius parts sunt sex, & sua cuiusque capita)

(243)

Œconomica

A Latin MS. is Dresd. Db 92, 93 ; s. xv, f. 16b (trans. ab Armengando Blazii de Arabico in Latinum. Inc. Omnis domus regimen. Expl. et timeat eos)

(244)

Ad Paternum

Latin MSS.

Chartres : Autricens. 62 (115) ; s. x, f. 54 (Alfabetum ad Paternum. Inc. I, ter ustum fit maxime de clavis cupreis. Expl. ad factum stiptica est. Explicit qualitas omnium herbarum)

Munich : Monac. 11343 (Polling. 43) ; s. xiii, f. 4 (Gal. Dogma ad Paternum)

Rome : Palat. 187 ; s. viii, f. 9 (Similar to Autricens. 62)

(245)

De peste

Latin translations

— Jo. Bapt. van Helmont. Opus. med. inaudit. de inaudit. de
febribus, de humoribus, Gal. lib. de peste. Amsterdam, 1648.

— See EHRHART (B.). Resp Commentarius . . . in historiam
Galeni de Peste. 1661. 4° *1179 d. 4 (11)* [B.M.]

(246)

De plantis

Latin MSS.

Paris : Parisin. 6837 ; s. xiv (De qualitate herbarum et
aromatum)

11219 ; s. ix, f. 207

Rome : Barberin. IX 29=767 ; s. —, f. 267 (Liber ad
Patricium missus de qualit. herbarum
et aromatum)

Palat. 1100 ; s. —, f. 1

Vatic. 2388 ; s. —, f. 84

4417 ; s. —, f. 96–8 (Palomia de pigmentis et
herbis.   Inc. Pro liquaceo mittes
agate)

4422 ; s. —, f. 1

(247)

De pica, vitioso appetitu, ex Galeno per Aëtium

Latin translations

— Chart. VII, p. 873

(248)

De causis procatarticis

Inc. Antiqui quidem physicorum
Expl. dicat videre nos nihil.

Latin MSS.

Dresden : Dresd. Db. 92, 93 ; s. xv, f. 445a

Paris : Parisin. 6865 ; s. xiv, f. 6b

Latin translations

— D. II, f. 17 (Nicolao de Regio interpr.)

— C. II, f. 491 (Inscr. Cl. Gal. De causis procatarticis Liber, ad Gorgiam, in quatuor capita distinctus ; quorum argumenta non apposuimus, quod parum Latina, ideoq ; hæc translatio, Græcum exemplar excusum non extet.) Nicolao Regio Calabro Interprete.

(249)

De passionibus puerorum

A Latin MS. is at Florence [Laurent.-Leopold (Biscionian.) 10 ; s. xiv, f. 184b (Inc. Ut testatur Hippocrates. Expl. lumbricos mirifice interficit)]

(250)

Compendium pulsuum

Inc. Hoc ei quod de pulsibus

Expl. in arteriis perficitur in eo.

Latin MSS.

Breslau : Vratisl. bibl. univ. IV F 25 ; s. xiii, f. 161, 162 (De comparatione pulsus sec. diastolen et systolen= Gal. comp. puls.)

Cesena : Malatest. D XXV, 2 ; s. xiii (De compendiositate pulsuum seu synopsis librorum de pulsibus)

Leipzig   Lipsiens. bibl. univ. Repos. med. I 4 ; s. — (Commentum pulsuum)

Munich : Monac. 490 ; a. 1488–1503 (De compendiositate ipsius pulsus interpr. Burgundione)

Oxford : Coll. Balliol. 231 ; s. xiv in. post f. 206b

Paris : Parisin.   6865 ; s. xiv, f. 138c

15455 ; s. xiii, f. 178

Rome : Palat. 1094 ; s. xiv, f. 547

1099 ; s. xv, f. 60

Urbin. 247 ; s. xiv, f. 252

Vatic. 2375 ; s. xiv, f. 271 (De compendiositate pulsus. Inc. Pulsus igitur diastole)

2376 ; s. —, f. 113

2378 ; s. —, f. 102

2383 ; s. —, f. 134

Latin translations

— D. I, f. 102

— C. IV, f. 1029 (Cl. Gal. Adscriptus Liber, Cui Titulus est, Compendium Pulsuum). Anon. Interpr.

(251)

De sanguine et flegmate

Latin MSS.

Brussels : Bruxell. 3701–15 ; s. f. 2 (Inc. Sanguinis vero calodus. Expl. in arte medicorum)

Paris : Parisin. 11219 ; s. ix, f. 17 (Similar to Bruxell.)

(252)

Secreta

Arabic and Latin MSS. are known.

Latin MSS.

Basle : Basil. D III 1 ; s. —

D III 6 ; s. —

D III 8 ; s. —

Bourges : Biturigens. 299 (247) ; s. xiv, f. 97 (De secretis secretorum)

Cues : Bibl. Nic. Cusani med. 15 ; s. xiv, No. 4

Eton : Bibl. Coll. 132 ; s. xiii, No. 10 (De secretis)

Munich : Monac. 4119 (Aug. S. Cruc. 19) ; s. xiv, f. 723 (De sapone muscato Gal. id est de secretis secretorum)

13026 (Rat. civ. 26) ;. s. xiv, f. 1 (Liber de
secretis Gal. Inc. Ignis qui descendit
de cælo super altare. See De medicinis
experimentatis)

Oxford : Bodl. MSS. Angl. 2461 ; s. —

Coll. Corp. Christ. 125 ; s. xiv, xv, xiii, f. 78 (Super
Hermatis librum secretorum expositio. Inc.
Quoniam in quo philosophorum doctissimi
desudavere)

Regensburg : Bibl. Urb. 44 ; s. — (similar to Monac. 13026)

Rome : Palat. 1205 ; s. —, f. 33 (Gal. secreta et alia medica.
Inc. Dixit Galenus)

Seville : Bibl. Colombin. B B 150, 5 ; s. xv

Wolfenbüttel : Guelferbyt. 1014 (Helmst. 912) ; s. xv, f. 72–3

2156 (12. 4. Aug.) ; s. xv, f. 178–9
(Quattuordecim experi-
menta de secretis Gal. ad
amicum quendam)

Latin translations
— D. II, f. 198 [?]

(253)

Liber secretorum ad Monteum

Inc. Rogasti me, amice Montee
Expl. ad omne quod narravimus.

Latin MSS.

Berlin : Phillipps. 1672 (166) ; s. xiv, f. 26

Cambridge : Cantabr. St. Petri 33 ; s. xiii/xiv, f. 186c

Cesena : Malatest. D XXV 1 ; s. xiii, f. 155 (Secretorum liber)

Chartres : Autricens. 284 (340) ; s. xiii, f. 251

293 (351) ; s. xiv, f. 118

Erfurt : Amplon. F 249 ; s. xiii, f. 246

Escurial : Scorial. H. III. 2 ; s. xiv, f. 3 (Expl. alius liber ab
isto, transferam ipsum)

Leipzig : Lipsiens. bibl. univ. Repos. med. I 4 ; s. —
Madrid : Matrit. bibl. nac. 1410 (ol. L. 65) ; s. xiv, f. 193
Munich : Monac.   276 ; s. xiv, f. 76
              640 ; s. xv, f. 78
              12021 (Prüf. 21) ; a. 1440–7, f. 1 (Liber
                 secretorum)
Nürnberg : Ebnerian.   4°   91 ; s. —, No. 3 (Lib. secretor. qui
                 dicitur Antidotarius)
Oxford : Coll. Balliol. 231 ; s. xiv, in. f. 39b
Paris : Parisin.   7031 ; s. xv, No. 1
             7046 ; s. xiii, No. 2
             7831 (?).   [Probably a misprint, and
                 intended for 7031]
             15456 ; s. xiii, f. 157
Rome : Palat.   1094 ; s. xiv, f. 398
           1234 ; s. —, f. 261
     Urbin. : 247 ; s. xiv, f. 61
     Vatic. 2375 ; s. xiv, f. 505
            2385 ; s. —, f. 271 (Expl. turbit albi aur. Sine
               tit. tradit.)
            2414 ; s. —, f. 193
            4422 ; s. —, f. 9–25
            4471 ; s. —, f. 31
Wolfenbüttel :   Guerferbyt. 2841 (83. 7. Aug.) ; a. 1432,
              f. 98–107

Latin translations
— D. II, f. 198
— C. IV, f. 1137 (Inc. Rogasti me, amice Montee. Expl.
transfera ipsum). This translation, which is anonymous, consists
of seventy-four chapters.

(254)

De cura senectutis

A Latin MS. is at Oxford (Bibl. Ædis Christi n. 1592).

(255)

De situ regionem

Latin MSS.

Madrid : Matrit. bibl. nac. 1978 (ol. L. 60) ; s. xiv, f. 95 (Inc.
Situm regionis an sit in vallem vel in montes.
Expl. deinde calida et sicca)

Oxford : Laudian. Misc. 617* ; s. xv, f. 289 (Ex Gal. libro de
sit reg. et temporum constitutione)

(256)

De spermate

Inc. Sperma hominis descendit
Expl. terra vertitur in humiditatem.

Latin MSS.

Basle : Basil. D III 8 ; s. — (De XII portis medicinæ
microtechn.)

Bourges : Biturigens. 299 (247) ; s. xiv, f. 91 (Microtegni, i.e. liber de spermate seu de XII portis)
[See Sections 160 and 189]

Cambridge : Cantabr. Caius Coll. 345 ; s. xiv, f. 46 (Micro-
tegni. Expl. per naturam sui corporis)
St. Petri 33, s. xiii/xiv, f. 119b (Inscr. Similar to
Biturigens. 299)

Cesena : Malatest. D XXV 1 ; s. xiii, f. 162
D XXV 2 ; s. xiii
S V 4 ; s. xiv, f. 48
S XXVI 4 ; s. xiii, f. 42

Chartres : Autricens. 284 (340) ; s. xiii, f. 247
293 (351) ; s. xiv, f. 123

Erfurt : Amplon. F 249 ; s. xiii, f. 253 (Inscr. resembles that
of Biturigens. 299. Expl. similar to
Cantabr. Caii 345)

F 278 ; s. xiv in. f. 78 (Inscr. resembles
that of Biturigens. 299. Expl. ex qua
acuitione et calore)

Eton : Bibl. Coll. 132 ; s. xiii, No. 11 (De spermate vel de XII
portis)

London : Addit. (Br. Mus.) 18, 210 ; s. xiii, xiv, f. 123 (Microtegni)

Lambethan. 244 ; s. xv, f. 30 (Microtegni de XII
portis)

Marburg : Bibl. Univ. B 2 ; s. xiii, f. 1 (Sine auctoris nomine)

Oxford : Coll. Balliol. 231 ; s. xiv, f. 34b (Microt. vel de
spermate) et f. 37 (De XII signis vel portis vel
microtegni. Inc. Sciendum quod XII sunt.
Expl. similar to Cantabr. Caii)

Paris : Parisin. 15456 ; s. xiii, f. 187 (Inscr. similar to
Biturigens)

Rome : Palat. 1094 ; s. xiv, f. 392

1298 ; s. —, f. 226 (Macrotegn. seu Microt.)

Urbin. 246 (ol. 457) ; s. xiv, f. 192 (Expl. capilli
tendunt in subedinem)

Vatic. 2383 ; s. —, f. 44

Latin translations

— D. I, f. 38

— C. IV, f. 925 (Inscr. Cl. Gal. Adscriptus Liber De Spermate
Inc. Sperma hominis descendit. Expl. terra vertitur in humiditatem) Anon. Interpr.

(257)

Subfiguratio empirica

Inc. Omnes medici qui colunt empiriam
Expl. de dissonantia eorum dictum est.

A Latin MS. is Monac. 465 ; a. 1503, f. 80 (Apogr. libri Venetiis,
a. 1503 editi)

Latin translations
— D. II, f. 290 (Nicolao de Regio interpr.)
— C. V, Isag. f. 101 (Incerto Interprete)

(258)

De vinis

Inc. Vinum aquosum nominant homines
Expl. utuntur antiquiores ad antidota.

Latin MSS.
Cesena : Malatest. S V 4 ; s. xiv, f. 41
      S XXVI 4 ; s. xiii, f. 34
Paris : Parisin. 6865 ; s. xiv, f. 53d
     Nouv. acq. 343 ; s. xiii, f. 69
Rome : Vatic. 2384 ; s. —, f. 29
     2386 ; s. —, f. 143

Latin translations
— D. I, f. 127
— C. IV, f. 1067 (Anon. Interpr.). Inc. and Expl. as stated
above.

(259)

Vocalium instrumentorum dissectio

Latin translations
— Chart. IV, p. 219
— Junt. VII, inter frgm. Gal. f. 48
— Claudii Galeni aliquot opuscula &c. 1550. 8° De
vocalium instrumentorum dissectione A. Gadaldino interprete.
540 d. 12 [B.M.]

(260)

De voce et angelitu

Inc. Si nervis qui sunt inter costas
Expl. medius inter voluntatem et naturam.

Latin MSS.
Breslau : Vratisl. bibl. univ. IV F 25 ; s. xiii, f. 94

Cambridge : Cantabr. St. Petri 33 ; s. xiii/xiv, f. 167b

Cesena : Malatest. D XXIII 1 ; s. xiii

       S V 4 ; s. xiv, f. 47 (De voce)

Chartres : Autricens. 284 (340) ; s. xiii, f. 138

Dresden : Dresd. Db 92, 93 ; s. xv, f. 24c

Erfurt : Amplon. F 249 ; s. xiii, f. 194

Eton : Bibl. Coll. 132 ; s. xiii, No. 8

Florence : Laurent. plut. 73, 11 ; s. xiv, f. 30 (De voce)

Montpellier : Montepess. (École de méd.) 18 ; s. xiii

Munich : Monacens. 276 ; s. xiv, f. 81 (De voce)

       640 ; s. xv (De voce)

Oxford : Coll. Balliol. 231 ; s. xiv, in. f. 55

Paris : Parisin. 15456 ; s. xiii, f. 186

      Nouv. acq. 343 ; s. xiii, f. 70

Rome : Palat.   1094 ; s. xiv, f. 211

      1097 ; s. —, f. 116

      1098 ; s. xv, f. 11

    Urbin.   235 ; s. xiv, f. 149

      247 ; s. xiv, f. 243

    Vatic.   2376 ; s. —, f. 114

      2378 ; s. —, f. 104

      2382 ; s. —, f. 63

      2383 ; s. —, f. 42

      2414 ; s. —, f. 192

Venice : Marcian. cl. XIV 6 ; s. xiv, f. 66, 67

Volterra : Volaterran. 103 (6365) ; s. xv, f. 85

Latin translations

—   D. I, f. 81

—   C. IV, f. 1013 (Anon. Interpr.)

(261)

De vulneribus

A Latin MS. is Monac. 264 ; a. 1380, f. 86 (" Exc. de vulneribus ex libro 1–6 Gal.") See Section (146)

(262)

In Hippocratem de septenario numero

Of the MSS. only the Arabic are known.   See Ch. 2 of this work.

(263)

De morte subita

Of the MSS. a single Arabic manuscript is known. See Ch. 2 of this work.

(264)

De nominibus medicinalibus

Of the MSS. a single Arabic manuscript is known. The Arabic MS. is possibly the same as that mentioned by Kühn I, p. CXCII, " De vocibus in medica arte usitatis."

(265)

De secretis feminarum et virorum

Of the MSS. only the Arabic are known.

(266)

De prohibenda sepultura

Of the MSS. the Arabic and Hebrew are kncwn.

(267)

Excerpta varia

Under this head are shown a collection of Latin works, a number of which are known in the Greek manuscript.

Latin MSS.

Basle : Basil. D II 3 ; s. — (Præcepta de emendanda sanitate)
　　　　　　　D II 13 ; s. — (Sanitatis conservandæ regulæ)
Breslau : Vratisl. bibl. acad. Ac. III 9 4 ; s. xv, f. 206 (Breve compendium de melioribus dictis Gal. Avic. Hipp.)

Cambridge : Cantabr. Caius Coll. III ; s. xiv, f. 407
Douaneschingen : Fürstenb. Bibl. 798 ; s. xvii, f. 1 (Aphorismi
                Rabbi Moysis ex Gal. collecti)
Erfurt : Amplon. F 259 ; a. 1408, f. 63 (Exempla ex operibus
             Gal. . . . nova extracta)
Erlangen : Bibl. Univ. 1089 ; s. xvi (Catechismus artis medicæ
                        ex doctrina Hipp. Aristot.
                        Gal. alior.)
              1106 ; a. 1597 (Loci communes operum
                        Hipp. menon etiam Gal. in
                        quibusdam explanationes)
Florence : Laurent. plut. 29, 8 ; s. xiv, f. 25
Jena : Bibl. acad. 116 ; s. —, No. 4 (Tract. ex libro Alpachimi
          et sentent. Hermatio collectus)
Leipzig : Lipsiens. bibl. univ. Repos. med. II 43 ; s. —(Tabula
          Gal. medicinalis)
Marburg : Bibl. Univ. B 14 ; s. xv, f. 97 (Inc. Iam Galenus
            ostendit totum quod necessarium est serie)
Oxford : Coll. Corp. Christ. 261 ; s. xvi in. f. 149
       Coll. Merton. 324 ; s. xv, f. 1
       Coll. Univ. 118 ; s. —
Paris : Parisin. 6879 ; s. xvi, No. 1 (Loci communes ord.
             alphab.)
           7831 ; s. — (Selecta e Gal. de variis morbis
               remediis que). This MS. possibly
               should read 7031, see " Liber
               secretorum ad Monteum "
          11218 ; s. ix, f. 42
Reichman : Bibl. d. Benediktinerabtei (Collectio aphorismor.
          ex Hipp. et Gal.)
Rome : Palat. 226 ; s. xv, f. 117
          398 ; s. xv, f. 1
        1091 ; s. —, f. 1

1205 ; s. —, f. 33 (Secreta et alia medica)

1211 ; s. — (Opera varia)

Vatic. 2376 ; s. —, f. 89–90 (Inc. Postquam incepi
. . . meos simplices in meo libro
declarari. Expl. in illis quæ sunt
meliora tres)

4417 ; s. —, f. 115–8

Subiaco : nr. 59 ; s. xiii, f. 22 (Inc. Summæ quæ sunt in
sermone primi libri Gal.)

Utrecht : Traiectan. Bibl. Univ. 688 ; s. xiv/xv, f. 81–5 (Ex
libris Hipp. et Gal.)

Venice : Marcian. cl. X 156 ; s. xiv, f. 57

Wolfenbüttel : Guelferbyt. 2189 (16. 3. Aug.) ; a. 1440–4,
f. 210–258ᵛ (Mundini Foroiuliens, synonyma
satis certa, longa et multa, sec. Gal.)

(268)

Indices in Galenum

Greek and Latin MSS. are known. A Latin MS. is Cantabr.
Caius Coll. 98 ; s. xv, f. 215 (Tabula librorum Gal. Inc. Abstentia.
Expl. imperf. in littera G.)

(269)

Laterculi librorum Galeni antiqui

Arabic and Latin MSS. are known. The Arabic MS. is the
work of Ḥunayn ibn Isḥāq (see Ch. 2 of this work).

Latin MSS.

Eton : Bibl. Coll. 127 ; s. xiv, f. 271b (Gal. opera recensentur)

Montecassino : Casinens 397 ; s. xiv, f. 50ᵛ (Inscr. Con-
numeratio librorum Galeini. Inc. G.
promiserat se numerum librorum morum
ostensuram)

Note.—The Arabic MS. is the work of Ḥunayn (Johannitius).

(270)

Scholia in Galenum

Greek and Latin MSS. are known. A Latin manuscript is
Douai ; nr. 717 ; s. xvi (Scholia in Hipp. et Gal libros anatomicos)
Latin translations

— Ed. Basileæ, 1537. 8° *543 a. 2 (1)* [B.M.]

" Medicorum schola, hoc est, Claudii Galeni Isagoge, sive
Medicus " [J. Guinterio interprete]

(271)

Isagogici Libri

A collection of Latin works which came to be known by this
name during the Middle Ages (See Gal. op. ed. Lugduni, 1550,
tome 5 . . . Elenchus Librorum Galeni omnium, qui in hoc opere
continentur).

The following constituted the " Isagoge " of Galen :—

Oratio suasoria ad artes, a Ludouico Bellisario medico
　　Mutinensi Latinitate donata . . . columna 　 5
Si quis optimus medicus est, eundum esse philosophum
　　eodum interprete 17
De sophismatis in verbo contingentibus, liber ab Horatio
　　Limano translatus 21
Quod qualitates incorporeæ sint, liber, eodem interprete 25
De libris propriis liber, a Joanne Fichardo Francofordiano
　　Latinitate donatus 33
De ordine librorum suorum, ab eodem Latinus factus . 47
De sectis, ad eos, qui introducuntur, a Ludouico Bellisaric
　　Latinus factus 51
De optima secta liber, Junio Paulo Crasso Patauino inter-
　　prete 55
De optimo docendi genere, Erasmo Roterodamo interprete 97
De subfiguratione empirica, incerto interprete . . . 101

De constitutione artis medicæ, liber, a Bartholomæo Sylvanio
    translatus 113
Definitiones medicæ : ab eodem itidem tranductæ . . 135
Introductio, seu Medicus, ab Joanne Andernaco Latinus
    factus 159
Quomodo morborum simulantes sint de depræhendendi,
    Joanne Fichardo Francofordiano interprete, recognitus 195
Ars medicinalis, Nicolao Lecniceno, interprete . . 199

(272)

Galeni Opera

This section consists of a catalogue of the Galenic works in the British Museum. The list is limited to only those editions that are meant to represent the works of Galen as a whole, and are confined to the Latin editions in the British Museum.

The details given are—the title of the work, a note on the contents of the volumes, the names of the principal translators, the editors (if known), place and date of publication, the index number in the British Museum Catalogue, and a note on the volumes, e.g. title page, pagination, index, &c.

The main body of the works here described, it will be noted, is compiled from " late translations ", and show Galen with the præ-nomen *Claudius*, which is an invention of the Renaissance (Cf. K. Sudhoff : Geschichte d. Medizin, Berlin, 1922, p. 108, and L. Thorndike : History of Magic and Experimental Science, Macmillan, 1923, Vol. I, p. 122).

— Magni Hippocratis Coi et Claudii Galeni . . . universa quæ extant opera &c. *See* Hippocrates—Magni Hippocratis . . . opera &c. 1639 fol. *C. 48 l. 1*

— Hippocratis . . . et Claudii Galeni Opera . . . Græce et Latine &c. *See* Hippocrates—Magni Hippocratis . . . opera

&c. Paris, 1679 fol. Ed. Renatus Charterius, apud Pralard. *683 l. 1–13*

— Galeni operum omnium sectio prima (–octava) libros omnes Spurios Galeno attributos comprehendens. [Translated into Latin by D. Erasmus, F. Balamius and others.] (Oribasii de musculorum dissectione ex Galeno J. P. Crasso interprete.) Accesserunt . . . adnotationes . . . A. Ricco . . . authore. [Edited by A. Liccus and V. Trincavellius.] 10 Vol.

Apud Joannem de Farris &c. Venetiis 1541–44–42–44–41–44–45–44–43. 8° *540 c. 1–10*

Vol. VI is in two parts, the second being separately paged. This copy is imperfect, leaves D. III, D. VI, N. III, N. VI of part 2, Vol. VI and leaves R.L. VIII. Vol. VII being supplied in MS.

— Omnia Claudii Galeni . . . opera quotquot apud Græcos in hunc usque diem extiterunt. . . in Latinum linguam conversa . . . quibus præmissa est præfatio dedicatoria (by H. GEMUSÆUS) Medicine primam inventionem ejus incrementa, tum ipsam quo Galeni vitam . . . depigens. Duplex . . . adjectus est index &c.

Copious MS. notes [by J. Cornarius]. 8 tom. in 9 pt.

Per Hier. Frobenium et Nic. Episcopium ; Basileæ, 1542 fol. *774 N. 13*

The index forms a separate part of tom. 8

— Claudio Galeni Pergameni omnia tum quæ antehac extabant, tum quæ nunc primum inventa sunt, opera ; in Latinam linguam conversa (by L. Bellisarius and others) emendata, et integritati restituta (Præfatio J. Montani, digestionis librorum Galeni rationem docens. Hippocratis De ære, aquis, et locis libellus, J. Cornario interprete. De laqueis, Oribasii, liber ex Heracle. De melancholia ex Galeno Rufo, et Possidonio, ab Ætio conscripta, J. Cornario interp. Oribasii de cucurbitulis, scarificationibus &c. A. Gadaldino interprete. Oribasius ex Heliodoro de machinamentis. V. Vidio interprete.) Accesserunt capitum numeri et argumenta . . . per C. Gesnerum. Adjectus est . . . index &c. 4 tom. Apud Joannem Frellonium ; Lugduni, 1550 fol.[1] *5401. 1–4*

Tom. 1 is in two parts, part 2 having a separate title-page and pagination ; tom. 4 is in three parts, part 2 having a separate title-page and pagination ; part 3 consisting of the index, has a separate title-page, and is without pagination.

— Another edition. Claudii Galeni . . . omnia, quæ extant (Galeno ascripti libri &c.) in Latinum sermonem conversa (by L. Bellisarius and others). (Hippocratis de ære, aquis et locis lib. J. Cornario interprete. Oribasii de cucurbitulis, scarificatione &c. A. Gadaldino interprete.) Quibus post summam antea adhibitam diligentiam, multum nunc quoque splendoris accessit, quod loca quam plurima ex emendatorum exemplarium collatione et illustrata fuerunt et castigata. His accedunt nunc primum C. Gesneri præfatio et prolegomena tripartita. De vita Galeni ejusque libris et interpretibus. (J. B. Montanus De ordine in

---

[1] The author is fortunately able to ' house ' a similar edition. This edition is unknown to Brunet and Deschamps. Graesse, III, 8 ; Jourdan, IV, 324, mentions only ed. Lyons 1552, in folio. The following is a note on the edition ' housed ' by the writer :—

" *Calenus. Opera.* Tomus Primus Operum Galeni, Complectens ea, quae ad corporis humani naturam, eiusque anatomen exquisite cognoscendam, pertinent. Adiectis quibus ad commodam victus rationem necessariis, Elenchum librorum post Joannis Baptistae Montani praefationem reperies. *Printer's mark.* Lugduni, apud Joannem Frellonium, M.D.L. *At end :* Lugduni, Excudebat Joannes Frellonius, M.D. XLVIII. *Folio. Rom. and Ital. char. with Greek passages.* 5 vols. in 5 . . . Vol V. Cl. Galeni Varia Opera, ac fragmenta, nunc primum inuenta, & Latino sermone donate . . . 6 ll. incl. title for : Cl. Galeni Pergameni, omnia tum quae antehac extabant, tum quae nunc primum inuen a sunt, Opera . . . Accesserunt capitum numeri, & Argumenta . . . per Conr. Gesnerum . . . *59 11 (numb. 236 cols.) incl. title for :* Operum Galeni Libri Isagogici Artis Medicae . . . + 1 *l. with colophon :* Lugduni, Excidebat Joannes Frellonius, Anno a Christo nato, M.D. XLIX. *A few diagrams in text. Large woodcut initials, some historiated, one in vol. I, leaf e⁴b, with portrait of Erasmus. Some parts waterstained, but otherwise a very good set ; in wooden bds., covered with Spanish brown morocco. Lyons, 1550."* This is the edition referred to in this volume as C. for reasons of brevity.

edendis legendisque Galeni operibus servando. Novus index in
. . . Galeni opera, bipartitus ; primus in legitima et genuina
[by S. Gratarolus] alter in spuria [by J. S. Stratander].)

Ex III officin : Frobenianæ editione. [Edited by C. Gesnerus.]
11 pt. MS. notes, partially effaced.

Per H. Frobenium et N. Episcopium, Basiliæ, 1562–61 fol.
540 l. 5–8

Parts 1–10 have each a separate title-page and pagination ;
part 11 has a separate title-page, and is without pagination.

— Theatrum Galeni, hoc est universæ medicinæ a . . .
Galeno diffuse sparsimque traditæ Promptuarium quo vel indicis
loco in omnes Galeni libros (of the Basle edition 1562) vel locorum
communium instar in re medica ; lector . . . utetur. A.
Mundellæ . . . Studio & labore . . . conditum & nunc demum
editum (by J. B. Mundella). Per Eusebium Episcopium &c. ;
Basileæ, 1568 fol. *540 l. 11*

— Claudii Galeni. Operum omnium Latinæ propediem
edendorum specimen [i.e. De optima corporis nostri constitution.
De plenitudine. De inæquali intemperie. Quomodo simulantes
morbum sunt depregendi. De ptisana]. Ex J. Lalamantii
recognitione, et castigatione Græci codicis . . . Ejus-dem
Lalamantii de ptisana sui temporis libellus.

Apud Petrum Santandreum : Genevæ 1579. 8° *540 d. 7 (5)*

— Galeni librorum quinta (–sexta) classis [translated by
T. Gerardus and others]. Sexta hac nostra editione non parum
ornamenti adepta ; locis pluribus quam in aliis superioribus
editionibus . . . emendatis (by J. Costæus) &c. Apud Juntas :
Venetiis, 1586 fol. *40 f. 4*

Classis 1–5, 7, &c., are wanting.

— Galeni opera ex octava Juntarum editione (translated by
L. Bellisarius and others). (Spurii Galeno ascripta libri. Galeni
operum fragmenta ; quarta editio). (H. Mercurialis, J. B.
Montanus, de Galeni libris. Galeni vita. Omnium Galeni
operum synopsis, Lucii Carani opera et labore confecta. Oribasii

de cucurbitulis, scarificatione &c. Sermo : de Laqueis ex
Heracle : ex Heliodoro de Machinamentis ; A. Gadaldino
interprete. De Diæta Hippocratis in morbis acutis ab
A. Gadaldino translatus. A. M. Brasavoli Index.) [Edited
by F. Paulinus.] 13 pt. Apud Juntas ; Venetiis. 1609 fol.
540 k. 1–5

Part 1 is without pagination ; parts 2–13 have each a separate
title-page and pagination.

— Another copy. *40 f. 1*

— Galeni opera ex nona Juntarum editione. [Translated by
L. Bellisarius and others. Edited by F. Paulinus.] (H. Mercurialis
. . . de Galeni libris. Galeni vita, nunc recognita et . . .
adnotationibus aucta. A. M. Brasavoli . . . [assisted by J. A.
Bonus] index . . . in omnes Galeni libros qui ex nona Junctarum
editione extant.) 13 parts.

Apud Juntas : Venetiis, 1625 fol. *540 k. 6–13*

Works—Epitome

— Speculum Galeni. Epitome Galeni, sive Galenus
abreviatus vel insisus aut intersectus que cunq. in speculo domini
Simphoriani Champerii cotinebatur apprehedens. Cui plurima
variarim traductionu eide in fine duplicata novaq. annectatur
Galeni opera cu. argumentis ejus-dem domini simphoriani.
Medicine ppugnaculu domini Simphoriani Chaperii . . . in
speculu medicine Galeni. Libri superadditi . . . Galeni vita
(A . . . S. chaperio . . . composita). De elementis Galeni
epithoma. De generatione animalium epithoma. De passione
unius cujusq. particule corporis cura ipsarum qui liber decem
tractatuu sive myamir intitulatur epithoma. Silve febrium ex
libris Galeni ad complementum libri myamir.

De dinamidiis liber. De morbis oculor. Galeni libri duo &c.
2 pt. G.L.

Symon Vincent : Lyons, 1512. 8° *540 b. 18*

Part 2 has a separate numeration, extending to leaf 35 ; the 59 leaves following are without numeration.

— Another edition. Speculum Galeni . . . Tabula . . . Constantini Aphricani terapetica seu megatechni super libros de ingenio sanitatis Galeni.

(Liber de oblivione a Costatino aphricano editus) 3 parts. G.L. Joannes de Jonvelle dictus piston ; Lugduni, 1517. 8° *732 bb. 37*

Register : part 1, sigs. a–s, part 2, aa–hh ; part 3 A–I, in eights, except sig. b, which has four leaves ; the pagination is continuous. There are three sheets (A.A.–C.C.) of preliminary matter.

— Epitome omnium Galeni . . . operum . . . per A. Lacunam . . . collecta. (Vita Galeni . . . ex Galeno ipso et ex variis authoribus per A. Lacuna . . . collecta. Cui accedit index locupletissimus &c. Annotationes in Galeni interpretes : quibus varii loci . . . et explicanturet . . . restituuntur, A. Lacuna . . . authore.)

Apud Hieronymum Cotum : Venetiis, 1548. 8° *540 C. 14*

Imperfect : wanting all except the " Vita Galeni ", the " Index ", and the " Annotationes ".

— Another edition. Epitomes omnium Galeni . . . operum. Postrema . . . hac editione quatuor opus-culorum . . . accessione locupletata. Vol. I. Lugduni, 1553. 16° *540 a. 1*

Imperfect wanting Vol. II–IV. The second leaf of the printer's epistle mutilated.

— Another edition. Epitome Galeni . . . operum per . . . A. Lacunam . . . collecta. (Galeni Pergameni vita . . . per A. Lacunam . . . collecta)

Basileæ, 1571 fol. *539 k. 11*

Another edition. Epitome Galeni operum . . . cum compendio ipsiusmet Galeni in Hippocratem, in calce hujus libri adjicto. Editio novissima. Lugduni, 1643 fol. *7320 h. 8*

(273)

Volumes in the British Museum Containing two or More Galenic Works in Latin Translation

The following contain two or more Galenic works, and constitute a complete list of such works [in Latin translation] in the British Museum. Against each of the publications is shown the works they contain, the names of the Latin translators, the place and date of publication (if known), and the number in the Index Catalogue of the British Museum.

Greek and Latin

— Medicorum schola, hoc est, Claudii Galeni Isagoge, sive Medicus (J. Guinterio interprete). Ejus-dem definitiorum medicinalium liber (Jona Philologo interprete). Basileæ, 1537. 8° *543 a. 2 (1)*

Imperfect wanting title-page and following leaf.

— Another copy. *540 b. 1*

Latin

— De inequali distemperantia. De bono corporis habitu. De confirmatione corporis humani. De presagitura. De presagio. De succidaneis. G. Valla . . . Interprete. Hoc in volumine hæc continentur ; Nicephori logica &c. 1498 fol. *1 B. 23982*

— Galeni opera N. Leoniceno interprete. De differetiis morboru. libri duo. De inequali intemperatura liber unus. De arte curativa ad Glaucone libri duo. De crisibus libri tres. Copious MS. notes. Per H. Stephanum ; Parisiis, 1514. 4° 540 f. 1 (1–4). Without pagination. Register a–t.

— Galeni Pergamensis de Temperamentis, et de Inæquali Intemperie libri tres, T. Linacro . . . interprete . . . Impressum . . . per J. Siberch, anno 1621.

Reproduced in exact facsimile, with an introduction by J. F. Payne and a portrait of T. Linacre. Macmillan and Bowes, Cambridge, 1881. 4° *1177 g. 36*

— Galeni Pergamensis de Temperamentis et de Inæquali Intemperie libri tres, T. Linacro interprete. MS. notes. Per Joannem Siberel, apud præclaram, Cantabrigiam, 1521. 4° *C. 31, e. 35 &c.* 82 leaves, the first 72 without numeration. Register A–S

— [Claudii Galeni Pergameni de motu musculorum libri duo N. Leoniceno interprete. (Galeni quos oporteat purgare medicamentis et quando)]

MS. notes. In ædibus Pynsonianis; Londini, 1522. 4° *C. 31 d. 9*

Only the last four leaves, commencing Sig. L. 3, and containing " Galeni quos oporteat purgare " &c.

— Comentum Galeni in Hippo. aforismos cum triplici interpretatione S. antiqua et Leoniceni ac Laurentiani. Hippocratis pnostic. Liber, cu comento Galeni fin tralatione antiqua. Ejus-dem prognostico. Liber, cum comento Galeni a Laurentiano in Latinam conversus. Ejusdem regiminis acutorum liber, cum comento Galeni; Galeni liber q. inscribit. Quos medicamentis purgari op. quos.

Prefatio N. Leoniceni in Librum techni Galeni. Galeni liber qui techni inscribitur, cu. quadruplici interpretatione, viz., Arabicæ, Latina antiqua et Leoniceniac. Laurentiani; cum comento HALY. Gentilis de Fulgineo Libellus, de divisione ordine librorum Galeni. N. Leoniceni Questio de trib. doctrinis ordinariis fin. siriam. Galeni. See Articella. Articella novissime per H. de Saliis recognita &c. 1523 fol. *539 h. 20*

— Galeni Pergameni de naturalibus facultatibus libri tres, T. Linacro Anglo interprete. (De decretoriis diebus.) Few MS. notes. In edibus R. Pynsoni; Londini, 1523. 4° *C. 31 e. 36*

— Galeni (Paraphrastæ Menodoti) . . . exhortatio ad bonas arteis, presertim medicinam; de optimo docendi genere; et quale oporteat esse medicu. D. Erasmo interprete. Apud J. Badium; Parisiis, 1526. 8° *540 d. 7 (3)*

— [Another edition] Galeni . . . Exhortatio &c. Apud Joan. Frob. Basileæ, 1526. 8° *774 d. 26*

— Galeni de temperamentis libri tres. De inæquali intemperie liber unus. T. Linacro interprete. London ? 1527. 8° *549 a. 5* Another edition of that printed in Cambridge, 1521. 4°

— Claudii Galeni de elementiis ex Hippocratis sententia libri duo. De optimo corporis humani Statu. De bono corporis habitu, Guinterio Joanne Andernaco interprete. MS. notes. Parisiis, 1528. 8° *540 b. 12 (1)*

— Claudii Pergameni de motu musculorum libri duo, N. Leonicene interprete. Nem libellus ejus-dem authoris, cui titulus est ; Quos oportet purgare, et qualibus medicamentis purgantibus, et quando. Parisiis, 1528. 8° *540 b. 13 (3)* Another edition of that printed in London in 1522. 4°

— Claudii Galeni . . . Introductio seu Medicus. De Sectis ad medicinæ candidatos opusculum. Guinterio Joanne Andernaco interprete. MS. notes. Parisiis, 1528. 8° *541 a. 9 (1)*

— Claudii Galeni . . . libri tres. Primus, de facultata naturalia, substantia. Secundus, q. animi mores, corporis temperaturam sequuntur. Tertius, de propriorum animi cujusq. affectuum ignitione et remedio. Guinterio Joanne Andernaco interprete. Parisiis, 1528. 8° *540 b. 13 (2)*

— Galeni . . . de naturalibus facultatibus libri tres. De pulsuum usu liber unus. Nem et quæ dem Pauli Æginetæ, de diebus criticis. T. Linacro . . . interprete. [Edited by J. Guinterius.] Few MS. notes. Paris, 1528. 8° *540 b. 13 (1)*

— C. G[aleni a]liquot libelli. (Quod animi mores corporis temperaturam seq. De viciis animi et eorum remedius. De sectis. Introductorius (Seu Medicus). De optima constitutione corporis humani. De plenitudine. De elementis. De atra bile. De tumoribus præter naturam) per Guinterium Joannem Andernacum partim recogniti, partim nunc primum versi. Few MS. notes. Basileæ. 1529. 4° *540 f. 3* The title-page is mutilated.

— C. Galeni Pergameni de atra bile liber. De tumoribus præternaturam liber. Guinterio Joanne Andernaco interprete. Parisiis, 1529. 8° *540 b. 12 (3)*

Dissectionis venarum arteriarumque commentarium. Ejus-dem de nervis compendium A. Fortolo interprete. Let. Basileæ, 1529. 18° *547 a. 3*

— Galeni opera de pulsibus H. Cruserio interprete.

[Containing the works : De pulsibus ad Tirones. De differ-entiis pulsuum. De dignoscendis pulsibus. De causis pulsuum. De præsigitura ex pulsibus. De usu pulsuum.]

Parisiis, 1532 fol. *539 k. 5 (1)*

— Claudii Galeni . . . de antidotis libri duo, a J. Guinterio . . . Latinitate donati. Ejus-dem Galeni de remediis paratu facilibus liber unus, eodem J. Guinterio interprete. Parisiis. 1533 fol. *539 k. 6*

— Claudii Galeni . . . de causis respirationis libellus. De usu respirationis liber unus. De Spirandi difficultate libri tres, J. Vasso interprete. Parisiis, 1533 fol. *539 k. 5 (2)*

— De pulsibus libellus ex Galeno collectus, et valuti in formulam redactus, in commoditatem rei medicæ candidatorum. Recens natus et editus, pp. 73. In officina C. Wecheli ; Parisiis, 1537. 4° *774 c. 2*

— Claudii Galeni de temperamentis libri III. De inæquali intemperie liber I. T. Linacro . . . interprete. Cum isagoge in eosdem libros, et scholiis marginalibus per J. Sylvium. MS. notes. Parisiis, 1537 fol. *543 g. 21 (2)*

Another edition of that published in Cambridge in 1521. A fragment : title-page and Sig. aa. II–IV only ; containing a commentary by Sylvius.

— Claudii Galeni . . . de curandi ratione per sanguinis missionem liber. Ejusdem de sanguisugis, revulsione, cucurbitula, et scarificatione tractatulus, Theodorico (Gerardo) Goudano interprete. Few MS. notes. Parisiis, 1539. 8° *540 d. 7 (1)*

— Erotematum . . . in libros de crisibus Galeni libri tres . . .

Galeni liber de ptisana. Galeni de eo quod sit animal id quod utero continetur.

De eo q. Galenus animam immortalem esse debitaverit, liber unus &c. See LUIS (A.) A. Ludovici . . . de Re Medica Opera &c. 1540 fol. *C. 54 k. 7 (3)*

— Claudii Galeni . . . introductio in pulsus ad Teuthoram, M. Gregorio interprete. Ejusdem de pulsuum usu. T. Linacro interprete. Few MS. notes. Apud Guliel. Rouillium ; Lugduni 1549. 16° pp. 94. *540 a. 6 (1)*

— Claudii Galeni . . . aliquot opera L. Fuchsio . . . Latinitate donata & commentariis illustratæ. De inæquali intemperie liber I. De differentiis & Causis morborum, sympto-matumque libri VI. De judiciis libri III. De curatione per sanguinis missionem liber I. (De temperamentis libri tres, de differentiis febrium libri duo. De laborantium locorum notitia libri VI.) 3 tom. MS. notes. Parisiis [1549–54] fol. *540 h. 2*

Tom. II is in two parts.

— Another copy of tom. I only *540 h. 1*

— Claudii Galeni aliquot opus-cula &c. (De musculorum dissectione . . . de nervorum dissectione . . . de vocalium instrumentorum dissectione ; A. Gadaldino interprete. Brevis denotatio dogmatum Hippocratis . . . C. Gesnero interprete. Galeni fragmentum ex quatuor commentariis quos ipse inscripsit, de iis quæ medicæ dicta sunt in Platonis Timeo, A. Gadaldino interprete. Principium commentarii primi, in primum librum Hippocratis epidemicorum, a N. Machello Latinitate donatum. Oribasii de cucurbitulis . . . A. Gadaldino interprete . . . Sermo, in septimo & octavo medicinalium collectionum ad Julianum Imperatorem Libro. Lugduni, 1550. 8° *540 d. 12*

— Claudii Galeni . . . de curatione per sanguinis missionem libellus. L. Fuchsio . . . authore. (Claudii Galeni . . . de hirudinibus, revulsione, cucurbitula et scarificatione libellus, L. Fuchsio interprete.) Lugduni, 1550. 8° *540 a. 10 (1)*

— Claudii Galeni . . . de naturalibus facultatibus libri tres, T. Linacro interprete. Huc accesserunt J. Sylvii (i.e. Du Bois) . . . cum scholia . . . tum epitome in eosdem libros . . . succinctis tabulis expressa.

Additusque est de naturalium facultata substantia liber, et an sanguis in arteriis natura contineatur, V. Trincabelio interprete ; omnia nunc demum . . . recognita. Lugduni, 1550. 8° *540 a. 6 (3)*

— Claudii Galeni . . . introductio in pulsus . . . De pulsuum usu. Lugduni, 1550. 8° *540 a. 6 (2)*

Another edition of that published in 1549.

— Galeni de ossibus ad tyrones. De nervorum, musculorum (A. Gadaldino interprete) venaru et arteriarum. (A. Fortolo interprete.) Vocaliu instrumentoru (A. Gadaldino interprete) Vulvæ (J. B. Feliciano interprete) dissectione libri. De motu musculorum libri duo (N. Leoniceno interprete). Adjecimus præterea Oribasii de musculorum dissectione libellum (J. P. Crasso interprete). Lugduni, 1551. 8° *540 a. 5 (2)*

— Claudii Galeni de constitutione artis medicæ (V. Trinca-velio interprete). De partibus artis medicæ (V. Trincavelio interprete). Introductio, seu medicus. Ars medicinalis (N. Leoniceno interprete). Lugduni, 1552. 8° *540 a. 14*

— De pulsibus libellus ex Galeni libris collectus. See GESNER (C.). Enchiridion rei medicæ triplicis. 1555. 8° *774 d. 1 (1–4)*

— Claudii Galeni opera aliquot (Galeni de propriis libris liber. De ordine librorum suorum liber. De ratione victus Hippocratis in morbis acutis. De decretis Hippocratis et Platonis liber primus), partim non ante ædita; partim emendata. See CAIUS (J.). J. Caii . . . opera aliquot et versiones &c. 1556. 8° *246 k. 6*

— F. Menæ . . . commentaria nuper edita in libros de sanguinis missione, et purgatione Claudii Galeni . . . quibus quid in era re aut agendum sit, aut adversantibus respondendum, utiliter admodum disceptatur. 2 parts. Ex officina Brocarii (Venice ?). 1558. 8° *540 b. 25 (1)*

— Claudii Galeni de facile parabilibus liber. De theriaca lib. II (J. Guinterio interprete). De antidotis lib. II (J. Guinterio interprete). De adumbrata figura empirici (D. Castello interprete). Lugduni, 1560. 8° *540 a. 15 (1)*

— Tomus primus commentarium in Claudii Galeni opera . . . complactens interpretationem Artis Medicæ, at librorum sex De locis affectis. [With the text, Lat.] Authore T. A. Veiga. 2 parts. Copious MS. notes. C. Plantin ; Antverpiæ. 1564–6 fol. *540 h. 13*

— Another copy. C. Plantin. Antverpiæ, 1564 fol. *539 k. 9* Imperfect : wanting the index to part 1, and title-page to part 2. With a variation in the preface, and with the addition to it of verses by J. Goropius Becanus.

— Claudii Galeni de alimentorum facultatibus lib. III. M. Gregorio interprete. De attenuante victus ratione, lib. I. eodem interprete. De bonis et malis succis, lib. I, F. Balamio interprete. De exercitatione parvæ pilæ libellus, J. Fichardo interprete. Lugduni. 1570. 8° *540 a. 16*

— L. Rogani . . . in Galeni libellum de pulsibus, ad Tyrones commentarius (with the text Lat.). In quo omnia, quæ Galenus XVI libris de pulsibus transegit, brevi exponuntur. Ejusdem de urinis libri tres ex Hippocrate & Galeno collecti. Edited by J. A. Maria. 2 parts. Vene tiis, 1575. 8° *1189 b. 7*

— Claudii Galeni . . . de differentiis febrium liber primus (secundiss). Interprete L. Laurentiano.

— De febribus curandis libri quinque, qui in his, qui de methodo medendo inscribuntur, sunt VIII, IX, X, XI, et XII. T. Linacro interprete . . .

De febribus curandis liber, qui primus est in his, qui de arte curativa ad Glauconem inscribuntur.

See FEBRES. De febribus opus sane aureum &c. 1576 fol. *776 m. 4*

— C. Galeni . . . 1. De optima corporis nosti constitutione. 2. De pleniore habitu. 3. De inæquali intemperie. 4. Quomodo simulantes morbum sunt deprehendendi. 5. De ptisana. Nem et J. Lalamantii de ptisana sui temporis libellus. Emendata . . . per eundem Lalamantium versio Latina &c. pp. 114. Autum ? 1578. 8° *540 b. 16*

— Galeni Ars Medicinalis illustrata commentariis F. Vallesii (F. Vallesii commentariola in libellum Galeni de inæquali intemperie.) Nuper recognita &c. Venetiis, 1591. 8° *540 b. 29* Imperfect : wanting pages 1–4

— F. Vallesii Cooarrubiani commentaria illustria in Claudii Galeni . . . libros subsequentes. I. Artem Medicinalem. II. De inæquali temperie libellum. III. Tertium de temperamentis librum. IV. Quinque priores de simplicium medicamentorum facultate libros. V. Duos de differentia febrium. VI. Sex de locis patientibus libros. (With the text Lat.)

Tractatus medicinales (by F. Vallesius). I. De urinis compendiaria tractatio. II. De pulsibus libellus. III. De febribus commentarius. IV. Methodi medendi libri tres. Omnia recens prima hac editione publicata, opera . . . J. P. Ayroldi, Marcellini &c. Coloniæ, 1594 fol. *540 L. 16*

— T. Roderici A. Veiga . . . opera omnia in Galeni libros edita, et commentariis in partes novem distinctis, expressa &c. [The " Ars Medica "—" De locis affectis "—and " De febrium differentiis " only. With the text . . . Præ superioribus editionibus eliminata &c.] Part I. Lugduni, 1594 fol. *539 k. 10*

— Claudii Galeni libellus de theriaca ad Pisonem, interprete et commentatore J. Juvene . . . Ejus-dem de antidotis lib. II ab A. Lacuna in epitomen redactii accessit epistola complectens medicamenta Bezoardica, quorum usus a peste præservat, auctore J. Juvene. Antverpiæ, 1595. 8° *549 a. 7*

— De temperamentis. De facultatibus naturalibus. [With a commentary.] See Segarra J. J. Segarræ . . . Commentarii Physiologici &c. 1596 fol. *540 h. 22*

— De pulsibus Tractatus . . . nunc denuo recogniti & aucti
&c. 2 parts. Venetiis, 1597. 8° *1189 b. 15*

The date of the colophon is 1575. A duplicate of the Venice
edition of that date, with new title pages; and some typographical
variations in the preliminary matter of part I.

— Menæ . . . commentaria in libros Galeni de Sanguinis
missione, et purgatione ; [with the text] quibus in hac editione
tertia additur. Libellus . . . de ratione permiscendi medicamenta
quæ passim in usum veniunt. Et. J. A. Lobeti . . . de foco
putredinis infebribus intermittentibus adversis termelium,
libellus hactenus non evulgatus. 3 parts. Augustæ Taurinorum
1625. 8° *540 b. 26*

Part 2 has a separate title page ; part 3 is separately paged.
Another edition of that published in Venice in 1558.

— Praxis medica curiosa. Hoc est Galeni methodi medendi
libri XIV. (Vita medica, hoc est Gelani ὑγιεινῶν, sive methodi
sanitatis tuendæ libri VI.) Nova . . . versione, et perpetuis
. . . commentariis et castigationibus illustrati a C. Hofmanno.
Adjectis nonnullis in Epidorpismatum vicem, cumprimis de
dieterio illo, medice viver esse pessime vivere. Cum oratione
J. G. Volckameri . . . Curante J. Scheffero. 3 parts Francofurti,
1680. 4° *541 C. 15*

— Miniaturea der lateinischen Galenos. Handschrift der
Kgl. Œffentl. Bibliothek. in Dresden, Db 92–3 in phototypischen
Reproduktion. Einleitung und Baschreibung von E. C. van
Leersum und W. Martin : pp. XXXVII, pl. 21, 1910. See Du
Rien (W. N.) Codices Græci et Latini photographice depicti &c.
Supplementum 8. 1897 &c. fol. *M.S. Facs. 147*

(274)

In Hippocratis Libros Diversos Commentarii

The following is a complete catalogue of the Latin translations
of Galen's Commentaries on the Hippocratic writings in the
British Museum. Galen being the main source of our knowledge

of medical literature after Hippocrates the works enumerated
hereunder are an excellent index of the medical views held regard-
ing the medicine of the ancients, by the medical scholastics of
the later Middle Ages. Against each work is given the index
number of the volume in the Catalogue of the British Museum.

— See Hippocrates—Works—Latin. Hippocratis opera
omnia, in que quidem Galeni commentaria hactenus Latio donata
&c. 1535. 8° *539 d. 1*

— See Hippocrates—Works—Greek & Latin : τοῦ μεγάλου
Ἱπποκράτους . . . τα εὑρισκόμενα . . . accessere variæ . . .
lectiones Græcæ . . . partim . . . Galeni commentariis . . . cum
Galeni Glossarum Hippocratis explicatione &c. Greek &
Latin. 1657 &c. fol. *434 k. 1*

— See Hippocrates. Two or more works. Greek and Latin.
Hippocratis Aphorismi . . . cum brevi expositione ex Galeni
commentariis desumpta. Ejusdem Hippocr. prænotionum libri
tres. Cum explanatione eodem ex fonte hausta per J. Butinum
1680. 8° *518 a. 42 (2)*

— See Hippocrates (Two or more works—Latin). Hippocratis
Aphorismi . . . Prædictiones cum Galeni commentariis &c.
1526. 8° *539 d. 7*

— 1527. 8° *539 d. 8*

— 1532 fol. *539 C. 2 (2)*

— See Hippocrates (two or more works—Latin). Hippocratis de natura humana liber, cum duobus commentariis
Galeni &c. 1539. 16° *539 a. 19 (1)*

— See Hippocrates. Two or more works—Latin. Hippocratis aphorismi . . . cum . . . expositione singulis aphorismis
ex Galeno supposita . . . Hippocratis prænotionum libri tres,
cum explanatione eodem ex fonte hausta &c. 1555. 8° *539 a. 4*

— See Hippocrates. Two or more works—Latin. Galeni
in Hippocratis librum de humoribus, commentarii tres ejusdem
reliquum sexti commentarii in sextum de vulgaribus morbis ;
itemque septimus et octavus &c. 1562. 8° *540 b. 8*

— See Hippocrates. Two or more works—Latin. H. Cardani in Hippocratis . . . prognostica opus . . . atque etiam in Galeni prognosticorum expositionem commentarii . . . Nem in libros Hippocratis de Septimestri et Octomestri partu et . . . in eorum Galeni commentaria, Cardani Commentarii &c. [With the text.] 1518 fol. *C. 79 f. 6 (1)*

— Epitome omnium rerum et sententiarum quæ annotatio dignæ in Commentariis Galeni in Hippocratem extant, per A. Lacunam . . . in Elenchum . . . digesta. Cui accessere nonulla Galeni Enantiomata per eundem A. Lacunam . . . collecta. Lugduni. 1554. 8° *539 d. 29*

— See Hippocrates. Prognostica. Prædictiones Hippocratis cum Galeni commentariis &c. Galeni in Hippocratis PRORRHE-TICI librum primum commentariorum libri tres &c. 1537. 8° *549 a. 6*

(275)

OTHER LATIN WORKS IN THE BRITISH MUSEUM CONTAINING REFERENCES TO THE GALENIC WRITINGS

This section contains the remainder of the Latin translations of the works attributed to Galen or commentaries thereon, that are to be seen in the British Museum. Against each of the works, is a note showing the main reference in the Index Catalogue of the British Museum. The name of the translator, the work or works, the year of publication, a description of the volume and the Index number.

———

— See ACCORAMBONIUS (F.) F. Accorambonii Interpretatio obscuriorum locorum . . . operum Aristotalis . . . contro-versiarum quæ versantur inter Platonicos, Galenum, et Aristo-telen examinatio &c. 1590 fol. *520 k. 14*

— See ACCORAMBONIUS (F.) Vera mens Aristotelis . . . Controversiæ item quæ sunt inter Platonicos, Aristotelcios, et Galenum examinantur &c. 1603 fol. *C. 76 g. 5*

— See ALBERTUS (Aloysius)   De nutritione argumento & generatione disputationes, in quibus Aristoteles defenditur adversus Galenum. 1627.   4°   *784 d. 11 (1)*

— See ALEXANDRINUS (J.)   Galeni Enantiomaton aliquot liber J. Alexandrino autore. Ejusdem Galeni encomium. 1548. 8°   *540 b. 23*

— See ALEXANDRINUS (J.)   J. Alexandrini Antargenterica pro Galeno. 1552.   4°   *539 e. 33*

— See ALEXANDRINUS (J.)   J. Alexandrini in Galeni præcipu scripta annotationes &c. 1581 fol.   *539 k. 12*

— See ALTOMARI (D.A. AB.)   De alteratione, concoctione . . . ex Hippocratis & Galeni sententia methodus. 1547. 8°   *540 b. 20 (2)*

— 1548.   16°   *540 a. 22 (3)*

— See AMATUS (J. C.)   Fructus Medicinæ, ex variis Galeni locis decerptii. 1623.   12°   *774 c. 9 '*

— See APOLLONIUS (Citiensis) Apollonii Citiensis et . . . aliorum, Scholia in Hippocratem et Galenum &c. 1834. 8° *540 e. 22*

— Anthologia anatomica ex scitis Galeni. [See Aristotle —Works—Greek & Latin] Aristotelis opera omnia &c. 1619 fol. *677 k. 2, 3*

— 1629 fol.   *29 h. 5–8*

— See BALLONIUS (G.)   G. Ballonii opuscula medica . . . In quibus omnibus Galeni et Veterum authoritas contra. T. Fernelium defenditur &c. 1643.   4°   *779 h. 3 (2)*

— See BEROALDUS (Philippus) the Elder. Opus-culum . . . De terremotu & pestilentia, cum annotamentis Galeni &c. 1510.   4°   *C. 37 f. 33 (3)*

— See BEROALDUS (P.) the Elder. Opusculum de terre motu . . . cum annotamentis Galeni. 1505.   8°   *541 e. 22 (1)*

— Another edition. See BEREOALDUS (P.) the Elder. Varia P. Beroaldi opus-cula &c. 1513.   4°   *1073 l. 5*

— 1515.   4°   *1073 l. 6*

— See BERTOTIUS (A.) Methodus generalis et compendiaria ex Hippocratis, Galeni et Avicennæ placitis deprompta &c. 1556. 8° *540 b. 33*

— 1558. 8° *545 a. 4*

— 1608. 8° *775 b. 11*

— See BOCCALINI (G. F.) Apologia adversus aliquot Donat Mutii in Hippocratem et Galenum con vitia &c. 1549. 4° *539 f. 6*

— See CAMUTIUS (A.) A. Camutii disputationes quibus H. Cardani conclusiones infirmantus, Galenus ab ejusdem injuria vindicatur &c. 1363.[1] 6° *774 b. 9 (3)*

— See CHAMPIER (S.) Cathegorie Medicinales . . . S. Chaperii . . . in libros demonstrationum Galeni Cathegorie Medicinales &c. 1516. 8° *7320 a. 8*

— See CHAMPIER (S.) Cribatio . . . & annatometa in Galeni . . . opera. 1516. 8° *774 b. 9 (1)*

— See CHAMPIER (S.) Symphonia . . . Galeni cum Hippocrate &c. . . . 1516. 8° *539 d. 27*

— 1528. 8° *774 b. 9 (2)*

— See CRATO (J.) J. Cratonis ad Artem medicam Isagoge. Additæ sunt in libros Galeni De Elementis, De Natura Humana &c. Periochæ J. B. Montani; cum epistola J. Cratonis, qua recte Galenum legendi ratio berviter ostenditus. 1560. 8° *540 b. 14 (2)*

— See CRATO (J.) Methodus θεραπευτική, ex sententia Galeni &c. 1555. 8° *1169 b. 1 (1)*

— See CREMONINI (C.) Apologia dictorum Aristotelis decalido innato adversus Galenum. 1626. 8° *543 b. 20 (6)*

— See CREMONINI (C.) Apologia dictorum Aristotelis de origine et principatu membrorum, adversus Galenum. 1627 fol. *C. 74 d. 7*

— See CUNÆUS (G.) G. Cunei apologiæ F. Putei pro Galeno in anatome examen. 1564. 4° *548 i. 2 (2)*

[1] *Sic.* I have inspected the book and the date should be 1563.

— See DIOSCORIDES (P.) Εὐπόριστα. P. Dioscoridis . . . adjectis symphonisi Galeni aliorumque &c. 1565. 8° *546 e. 15 (1)*

— See DONATIUS (J. B.) Commentationum medicarum liber IV, de judiciis quæ in Galeni voluminibus . . . desiderari videntur. 1580. 4° *540 e. 15 (1)*

— See DU BOIS (J.) In Hippocratis et Galeni physiologæ partem anatomicam isagoge &c. 1555 fol. *543 g. 21 (3)*

— See DU BOIS (J.) Morborum internorum prope omnian curatio . . . ex Galeno . . . selecta &c. 1545. 8° *776 b. 2 (1)*

— 1548. 8° *776 b. 2 (2)*

— 1549. 8° *776 b. 3 (1)*

— 1554. 8° *774 b. 17 (1)*

— See DU BOIS (J.) Ordo et ordinis ratio in legendis Hippocratis et Galeni libris.

1535 ? 8° *539 c. 11 (4)*

— 1561. 8° *539 b. 35 (2)*

— See DU CHESNE (J.) Apologia pro . . . Galeni medicina adversus Quercetani librum de priscorum philosophorum veræ medicinæ materia &c. 1603. 12° *547 a. 5 (1)*

— See DUNUS (T.) Muliebrium morborum . . . remedia ex . . . Galeno [and others] . . . collecta. 1565. 8° *456 h. 3 (2)*

— Elogium chronologicum [of Galen] auctore P. Labbeo. See FABRICIUS (JOHANN ALBERT) J. A. Fabricii . . . Bibliotheca Græca &c. Vol. 3. 1705 &c. *11852 C. 29*

— 1718 &c. *680 c. 1–14*

— 1790 &c. *2048 g*

— See FERRARIUS (O.) O. Ferrarii . . . de regulis medicinæ libri tres, ex Hippocrate, Galeno . . . collecti. 1566. 8° *540 b. 34 (1)*

— See FUCHS (L.) L. Fuchsii . . . de humani corporis fabrica ex Galeni et A. Vesalii libris concinnatæ, epitomes &c. 1551. 8° *548 c. 1*

— 1551 &c. 8° *548 c. 2*

— See GABRIEL, de Tarrega. Begin : Habes humane lector Gabrielis de Tarrega . . . opera brevissima . . . Textus Avicene . . . cum quisbusda. additionib. et concordatiis Galeni &c. 1524. 4° *542 f. 29 (1, 2)*

— See GRUNER (C. S.) Censura librorum Hippocrateorum, qua veri a falsis . . . segregantur. Collegit ex . . . Galeno . . . aliis–que . . . C. G. Gruner. 1772. 8° *539 e. 29*

— See GUINTERIUS (J.) Andernacus. Anatomicarum institutionum ex Galeni sententia libri IIII &c. 1539. 4° *541 c. 13 (2)*

— See HIPPOCRATES. [Two or more works—Latin.] De febribus commentarius, ex libris aliquot Hippocratis & Galeni . . . selectus &c. 1555. 8° *1166 c. 2*

— 1556. 8° *1166 d. 2 (1)*

— See Hippocrates [Coaca Præsagia] Magni Hippocratis Coaca Præsagia . . . brevi enarratione illustrata, decerpta a Galeno &c. Greek & Latin. 1657. 12° *539 a. 32*

— See HOFMANNUS (C.) C. Hofmanni . . . apologiæ pro Galeno . . . libri tres &c. 1668 4° *540 g. 10*

— See HERBST (W.) Philologist. Galeni Pergameni de Atticissantium Studiis testimonia &c. 1911. 8° *11313 g. 41*

— See HOFMANNUS (C.) C. Hofmanni de Thorace ejusque partibus commentarius . . . in quo discutiuntur præcipue et quæ inter Aristotelem et Galenum controversa sunt. 1627 fol. *548 k. 8 (2)*

— See HOFMANNUS (C.) C. Hofmanni Pathologia parva in qua methodus Galeni practica explicatur &c. 1640. 12° *775 d. 11*

— See HOFMANNUS (C.) C. Hofmanni pro veritate opellæ tres. Adrastea Galeni &c. 1647. 4° *542 f. 15*

— See HOFMANNUS (C.) C. Hofmanni Variarum Lectionum libri VI. In quibus loca multa . . . Galeni . . . explicantur. 1619. 8° *774 b. 25*

— See Hofmannus (C.)   Relatio historica judicii, accitin Campsis Elysiis . . . contra Galenum &c.   1642.   12° *1172 a. 5 (4)*

— Libellus de divisione librorum Galeni [by Gentilis de Fulgineo]   See Hunain ibn Ishak.   Begin : In hoc pclaro libro &c.   1487 fol. *540 k. 15*

— See Husain Ibn.   Abd Al-lah (Abu-Alz) called Ibn Sina, or Avicenna [Canon] Principis Avicennæ liber primus . . . Adjectis . . . interpretis scholiis Hippocratis et Galeni præcipue loca commonstrantibus.   1580.   4° *542 d. 1*

— See Introductio.   Introductio in vitalem philosophiam. Cui cohæret omnium morborum . . . additis . . . placitis . . . Galeni . . . explicatio &c.   1623.   4° *718 e. 37*

— See Jostreriis (J. de).   Admirationes medicæ ex doctrina Galeni . . . scilicet, de usu vesicantium promiscue in morbis omnibus &c.   1596.   4° *783 g. 12*

— Elogium.   See Labbe (P.)   Claudii Galeni Chronologicum Elogium &c.

— See Marinelli (C.)   De morbis nobilious animæ facultates obsidentibus libri tres . . . Quibus accedit liber patefaciens Galenum . . . Denique opusculum quoddam continens nonnulles controversias, inconstantias utque admirationes in dictis Galeni adimventus.   1615.   4° *776 c. 2 (1–3)*

— See Martini (G.)   Commentatiuncula in libri qui inscribitur de chymicorum cum Aristotelicis et Galenicis consensu ac dissensu caput XI, quod est de principiis chymicorum &c. 1621.   8° *1033 e. 10*

— See Martinus (Jacobus) of Dunkeld.   J. Martini Scoti . . . de prima simplicium et concretorum corporum generatione disputatio, in qua . . . Galeni & aliorum sententia de simplici et absoluta generatione proponitur &c.   1584.   8° *536 d. 16 (4)*

— See Massa (N.)   N. Massæ Epistolarum . . . tomus primus &c.   (Tomus alter . . . in quo multæ Galeni obscuræ enodantur sententiæ) tom. 2.   1558.   4° *1165 g. 3*

— See MONTANUS (C.) Comitis Montani . . . de morbis ex Galeni sententia libri quinque. 1580. 4° *544 f. 2*

— See MUNDELLA (A.) A. Mundellæ . . . Epistolæ Medicinales . . . in quibus . . . Galeni . . . loci obscuri . . . illustrantur &c. 1538. 8° *1165 b. 1*

— 1543. 4° *540 d. 34*

— See NANCEL (N. de) N. Nancelii . . . de immortalitate animæ velitatio adversus Galenum &c. 1587. 8° *774 b. 23 (1–2)*

— See ODDIS (M. de). De Morbi Natura et Essentia Tractatio . . . in qua . . . Hippocratis atque Galeni sententia defenditur. 1589. 4° *776 g. 1 (3)*

— See ODDIS (O. de) O. de Oddis . . . de pestis . . . curatione . . . apologia pro Galeno &c. 1570. 4° *1167 h. 3*

— See Oribasius. τὰ τῶν ᾽Οριβασίων ἰατρικῶν συναγωγῶν ἐκ τῶν Γαληνοῦ ἀνατομικά. Oribasii collectaneorum Artis Medicæ liber, quo totius corporis humani sectio explicatur, ex Galeni commentariis. Greek. 1556. 8° *1067 c. 21*

— See PERNICE (Ericus) Galeni de ponderibus et mensuris testimonia &c. 1888. 8° *8530 g. 40 (6)*

— See PICTORIUS (G.) Medicinæ tam simplices quam compositæ . . . ex Galeno &c. 1560. 8° *544 c. 39 (4–6)*

— See PONCE DE SANTA CRUZ (A.) In Avicennæ primam primi . . . tomus primus. (Disputationes de pulsibus, quibus Galeni et Avicennæ doctrina philosophice perpenditur). 1622 fol. *542 g. 14*

— See PUTEUS (F.) Physician. Apologia in anatome pro Galeno &c. 1562. 8° *540 c. 15*

— See RORARIUS (N.) Contradictiones . . . in libros . . . Galeni &c. 1572. 12° *774 b. 21*

— See RICIUS (P.) Pauli Ricii israhelite . . . copediu. quo . . . opostolica. veritate . . . plane cofirmat . . . Insuper quarti Tractat. exordio triplicem doctrine ordine. a Galieno obumbrate traditum perpulchre edit in lucem. 1507. 4° *4033 b. 66*

— See ROSENTHAL (H.)   De nervorum physiologia Galenica. Dissertatio historico-medica &c. 1848.   8°   *7385 a. 1 (9)*

— See RUDIUS (E.)   E. Rudii . . . liber de nima de anima, in quo probatur Galenum de vegetalis et sentientis animæ substantia reliquis omnibus rectius sensisse &c.   1611.   4° *549 d. 14*

— See SCALIGER (J.)   J. Scaligeri loci cujusdam Galeni difficilimi explanatio &c. 1619.   4°   *543 b. 19 (2)*

— See SENNERTUS (D.)   De Chymicorum cum Aristotelicis et Galenicis consensu ac dissensu liber I &c. 1619   8°   *1135 f. 25*

— See SERVETUS (M.)   Syruporum universa ratio, ad Galeni censuram diligentes expolita &c. 1537.   8°   *778 c. 41*

— 1546.   8°   *540 c. 21 (2)*

— See SERVETUS (M.)   Syruporum universa ratio, ad Galeni censuram . . . expolita &c. 1545.   8°   *547 c. 1 (1)*

— See SILVATICUS (M.)   Opus pandectarum Matthei Siluatici . . . cu. quotationibus auctoritatum Plenii Galenii alioru. auctor &c. 1499 fol.   *I. B. 22196*

— See SILVATICUS (J. B.)   Galeni historiæ medicinales a J. B. Silvatico . . . enarratæ. 1605 fol.   *539 k. 13*

— See SOCIO (N.)   De Temporibus et modis recte purgandi in morbis, tractatus ad . . . Galeni . . . scripta intelligenda necessarius &c. 1555.   8°   *1189 a. 25*

— See SPRACKLING (R.)   Medela Ignorantiæ.

— See SYLVANIUS (B.)   Index in librosom nes Galeni per Juntas Venetiis excusos. 1542 fol.   *540 i. 16*

— See THEOPHRASTUS [Two or more works] Θεοφάστου . . . περὶ ἰδρώτων . . . Libello de sudoribus adjecta sunt sudorum prognostica . . . Latinis versibus descripta, ex Hippocr.[atis] & Gal.[eni] scriptis. Greek & Latin. 1576.   8°   *539 d. 32 (3)*

— See TOLETUS (P. J.)   De methodo opus ad Galeni cætorumq. medicorum et philosophoru. libros (veluto claris) operiedos . . . necessaria. 1558.   4° *540 e. 13 (1)*

— See TRABONA (H.)   De Medicamento purgante quarta die

dissertatio. In qua cum Hippocratis tum Galeni auctoritatibus
. . . quarto die non esse purgandum statuitur. 1636. 8° 4°
1188 i. 2 (5)

— See TRISSINUS (A.) A. Trissini . . . problematum
medicinalium ex Galeni sententia libri sex. 1547. 8° *774 b. 15*

— See TRIVERIUS (J.) H. Thriveri . . . in . . . tres libros
Galeni de temperamentis et unum de inæquali intemperie . . .
commentarii quatuor &c. 1535. 4° *543 b. 20 (5)*

— De locis . . . pugnantibus apud Galeni Libellus. See
VALLES DE COVARRUBIAS (F.) Controversiarum medicarum . . .
F. Vallesii . . . editio tertia. 1591. 8° *775 e. 5*

— See VICARIUS (J. J. F.) Tractatus de intemperato
Hippocratico seu caco-chymiis Galeni &c. 1712. 4° *1033 l. 18 (1)*

— See VICTORIUS (B.) B. Victorii . . . de morbo Gallico
iber. Hinc annectitur de curatione pleuritidis per sanguinis
missionem liber ad Hippocratis & Galeni scopum. 1551. 8°
1174 b. 1

— See VOIGT (J. C. I.) Tractatus medicus . . . de passione
seu affectione hypochondriaca authoritatibus Galeni et Hippocratis suffultus &c. 1678. 4° *1191 k. 1 (4)*

— See ZALUZANSKY (A.) A. Zaluzanii . . . animadversionum
medicarum in Galenum et Avicennam libri VII. 1604. 8°
540 d. 19

— Claudii Galeni . . . Historiales Campi per D. S.
Campegium (i.e. Champier) . . . in quatuor libros congesti et
commentariis . . . illustrati. D. S. Campegii . . . Clysteriorum
Camporum secundum Galeni mentem libellus . . . Ejusdem de
phlebotomia libri duo. Basileæ, 1532 fol. *540 h. 10 (1)*

— Morborum internorum prope omnium curatio brevi
methodo comprehensa ex Galeno præcipue et M. Gattinaria per
J. Sylvium (i.e. Du Bois) selecta. Omnia nunc denuo in lucem
emissa. Copious MS. notes. Lugduni. 1548. 8° *545 a. 1 (1)*

— Vita Claudii Galeni ex propriis operibus collecta per
P. Labbeum. Parisiis, 1660. 8° *540 b. 21 (1)*

(276)

EDITIONS OF GALEN THAT ARE NOT IN THE BRITISH MUSEUM

Greek & Latin

Paris. [?]

Leipzig. 1821–33. 8° Ed. C. G. Kühn. In Officina libraria
      C. Cnoblochii

Latin

Venice. 1490. fol. per Philipp. Pintium de Caneto

Papiæ. 1516. fol. impr. per Jac. Paucidraoensem de Burgo-
      franco prid. Indus Junii

Venice. 1522. fol. expensis Luc. Ant. de giunta Florentini.

Ed. Juntina. 1528 (copy in the Vatican Library see Diels:
      Handscriften d. ant. Ärzte. 1, 2)

Venice. 1541. fol. ap. Juntas.

Lyons. 1552 fol. (mentioned by Jourdan IV 324).

Venice. 1562. fol. ap. Vinc. Valgrisium.

BIBLIOGRAPHY

The Caliphate

W. Muir : Annals of the Early Caliphate (1883).

The Caliphate, its Rise Decline, and Fall (1891).

S. Lane Poole : The Mahomedan Dynasties (1894).

C. C. Torrey : The History and Conquest of Egypt, North Africa, and Spain ; known as the Futūh Misr of Ibn Abd Al-Hakam. Edited from the Manuscripts in London, Paris, and Leyden by C. C. Torrey (New Haven and London).

E. Renaudot : Ancient Accounts of India and China, by two Mohammedan Travellers, who went to those parts in the ninth century, trans. from the Arabic (London, 1733).

Language and Literature

E. G. Browne : Literary History of Persia, vol. i (1902).

C. Huart : History of Arabic Literature (English translation by Lady M. Lloyd). Clement Huart's *Littérature arabe* may be read in the original series *Histoires des littératures* (Paris, 1912).

R. A. Nicholson : Literary History of the Arabs (1907).

Spain

H. E. Watts : Spain from the Moorish Conquest to the Fall of Granada (1893).

W. H. Prescott : History of Ferdinand and Isabella, ed. J. F. Kirk (1902).

A. H. Morejon : Historia de la medicina española, Madrid [Historia bibliografia, 7 vols., 1842–52].

Greek Medicine

Sir T. Clifford Allbutt : Greek Medicine in Rome, with other Historical Essays (Macmillan, 1921)

R. O. Moon : The Post-Hippocratic Schools of Medicine (The FitzPatrick Lectures, an Abstract), *British Medical Journal*, vol. i, 1923

C. Singer : Greek Biology and Greek Medicine (vol. i of Chapters in the History of Science. General editor, Charles Singer (Oxford, 1922)).

Arabian Medicine

F. Wüstenfeld : Die Academien der Araber und ihre Lehrer, 1837. Geschichte der Arabischen Ærzte und Naturforscher (Göttingen, 1840).

M. Steinschneider : Wissenschaft und Charlatanerie unter den Arabern im neunten Jahrhundert. Virchow's Arch. (Berlin, 1886).
Die europäischen Übersetzungen aus dem Arabischen (Vienna, 1904–5)

Max Simon : Sieben Bücher der Anatomie des Galen (Leipzig, 1906).

August Hirsch : Biographisches Lexikon der Hervorragenden Ærzte alter Zeiten und Völken (Vienna and Leipzig, 1884).

Albucasis : Liber Servitoris, liber xxviii (British Museum).

Johannes Channing : Albucasis de Chirurgia (Clarendon Press, 1778).

Mesuë opera, Venice, 1603 (British Museum).

Lucien Le Clerc : Histoire de la médecine arabe, 2 vols. (Paris, 1876).

Daniel Le Clerc : The History of Physick, English rendering by Drake & Baden (London, 1699).

K. Opitz : Die medizin im Koran (Stuttgart, 1906).

Alois Sprenger : De originibus medicinae arabiae sub Kalifatue (1840).

P. de Koning : Trois traités d'anatomie arabe (Leyden, 1903).

J. Amoreux : Essai historique et littéraire sur la médecine.

The (1001) Arabian Nights, ed. Macnaghton, vol. ii ; Sir R. Burton's translation, vol. v.

W. A. Greenhill : English translation of Rhazes' "Liber de variolis et morbillis" (Sydenham Society, London, 1848).

G. S. A. Ranking : The Life and Work of Rhazes, XVIIth International Congress of Medicine, 1913, section xxiii, History of Medicine, p. 237

E. G. Browne : Arabian Medicine [The FitzPatrick Lectures of 1919 and 1920] (Camb. Univ. Press, 1921).

Mediaeval Medicine

G. F. Fort : Medical Economy during the Middle Ages : a contribution to the history of European morals from the Roman Empire to 1400 (New York, 1883).

E. Dupouy : Le moyen âge medical (Paris, 1888).

H. M. Ferrari : Une Chaire de Médecine au XVe Siècle (Paris, 1899).

Sir T. C. Allbutt : Science and Mediaeval Thought (London, 1900).
The Historical Relations of Medicine and Surgery (London, 1905).

J. J. Walsh : The Popes and Science (New York, 1908).

M. Steinschneider : Die hebräischen Übersetzungen des Mittelalters (Berlin, 1893).

F. Wüstenfeld : Die Übersetzungen arabischer Werke in das Lateinische, xi Jahrhundert (Göttingen, 1877).

L. Choulant : Bûcherkunde für die Ältere Medizin (Leipzig, 1841).

C. Baeumker : Beiträge zur Geschichte der Philosophie des Mittelalters (Munster, 1916).

R. R. von Töply : Studien zur Geschichte der Anatomie im Mittelalter (Leipzig, 1898).

C. Singer : Science—" Medaeival Contributions to Modern Civilization " (Harrap, London, 1921).

D. Mackinnon : Scottish Collection of Gaelic MSS., XVII International Congress of Medicine, London, 1913, Hist. of Med., section xxiii.

The Incunabula

R. A. Peddie : Fifteenth Century Books, London, 1913. Conspectus incunabulorum, Pt. I (London, 1910).

W. L. Schreiber : Catalogue of illustrated incunabula (Leipzig, 1910–11).

General

W. G. Black : Folk-Medicine (London, 1883).

Sir E. Thorpe : Dictionary of Applied Chemistry, vol. i (London, 1921).

R. W. Livingstone : The Legacy of Greece (Clarendon Press, 1921).

Sir R. C. Jebb : Greek Literature (London, 1921).

Sir T. Clifford Allbutt : Science and Mediaeval Thought (Harvian Oration, 1900), *British Medical Journal,* 1900, vol. ii, pp. 1271–3.

De Lacy O'Leary : Arabic Thought and its place in History (Trubner's Oriental Series, 1922).

Charles Singer : Studies in the History and Method of Science (Oxford Univ. Press), vol. i, 1917, vol. ii, 1921.

Proceedings of the Royal Society of Medicine, 1917, vol. x, part ii.

Lister : *The Lancet,* 1867, vol. ii.

Johannes Freind : History of Physick, 2 parts (London, 1750).

Nicholson : Mystics of Islam (London, 1914).

Burckhardt : Civilization of the Period of the Renaissance in Italy, Eng. ed., 1890.

Camb. Modern History, vol. i (1902).

H. Osborn Taylor : The Mediaeval Mind, 2 vols. (Macmillan, 3rd ed., 1919).

R. R. Steele : The Secretum Secretorum Aristotelis in the works of Roger Bacon. [Opera hactenus inedita Rogeri Baconi, 1905–20.] The Mediaeval Panacea, Proc. of the Royal Soc. of Medicine, 1916, vol. x, part ii.

F. Hartmann : Die Literatur von Frûh- und Hochsalerno (Leipzig, 1919).

F. W. Putzger : Historischer Schul-Atlas (Leipzig, 1896).

K. P. Sprengel : Geschichte der Arzneikunde (Halle, 1792).

H. Diels : Die Handschriften der antiken Ärzte

    I. Teil. Hippokrates und Galenos. Aus den Abhandlungen der Königl. Preuss. Akademie der Wissenschaften von Jahre 1905. Berlin, 1905. Verlag der Königl. Akademie der Wissenschaften. In Kommission bei Georg Reimer.

    II. Teil. Die Übrigen Griechischen Ärzte ausser Hippokrates und Galenos. Berlin, 1906. In Kommission bei Georg Reimer.

The School of Salernum-Regimen Sanitatis Salernitanum. The English version, by Sir John Harington ; History of the School of Salernum by Francis R. Packard ; and a note on the Pre-History of the Regimen Sanitatis by F. H. Garrison (New York, 1920).

A. F. v. Schack : Poesie und Kunst der Araber in Spanien und Sizilien (Berlin, 1865).

W. Heyd : Geschichte des Levantehandels (Stuttgart, 1879).

D. Castelli : Il Commento di Sabbatai Donnolo sul libro della creazione (Florence, 1880).

N. Bubnov : Gerberti opera Mathematica (Berlin, 1899).

G. Voight : Die Wiederbelebung des classischen Alterthums (Berlin, 1881).

E. Renan : Averroës et l'Averroisme, 3rd ed. (Paris, 1866).

T. C. Wedel : The Mediaeval Attitude toward Astrology particularly in England (Yale Univ. Press, 1920).

F. H. Garrison : Introduction to the History of Medicine, 2nd ed. Saunders, 1917 (3rd ed. 1922).

T. Puschmann : History of Medical Education from the Most Remote to the Most Recent Times, translated and edited by E. H. Hare (London, 1891).

J. H. Baas : Outlines of the History of Medicine, translated and edited by H. E. Handerson (New York, 1889).

Robley Dunglison : History of Medicine, ed. by R. J. Dunglison (Philadelphia, 1872).

Roswell Park : Epitome of the History of Medicine (1897).

Max Neuburger : Gesch. d. Medizin (Stuttgart, 1908), English trans. by Ernest Playfair, vol. i (London, 1910).

E. T. Withington : Medical History from the Earliest Times (London, 1894).

H. I. Bull : The Bibliography of Bernard de Gordon's " De conservatione vitae humanae ", XVII International Congress of Medicine, London, Hist. of Med. (section xxiii).

O. Siren : Leonardo da Vinci (Stockholm, 1911).

Lewis Spence : Myths and Legends of Babylonia and Assyria (London, 1916).

The Encyclopædia Britannica, 11 edition (Cambridge Issue).

Hastings Rashdall : The Universities of Europe in the Middle Ages (Clarendon Press, 1895).

Sir R. Lodge : The Close of the Middle Ages (London, 1920).

Sir Wm. Osler : The Evolution of Modern Medicine (New Haven, 1921).

Aequanimitas, 2nd ed. (London, 1906).

Carl Brockelmann : Geschichte der arabischen Litteratur, vol. i (Weimar, 1898).

Galen : Opera Omnia, Lyons, ed., 1550.

Galen on the Natural Faculties, with an English translation by A. J. Brock (London, 1916).

Proceedings of the Third International Congress of the History of Medicine (London, 1922).

J. L. Heiberg : Mathematics and Physical Science in Classical Antiquity, Oxf. Univ. Press, 1922. (This is vol. 2 of " Chapters in the History of Science " edited by Charles Singer.)

K. Sudhoff : Geschichte der Medizin im Überblick mit Abbildungen (Jena, 1921).

Geschichte der Medizin, dritte und vierte Auflage von J. L. Pagel's " Einführung in die Geschichte der Medizin " (Berlin, 1922).

Lynn Thorndike : History of Magic and Experimental Science (Macmillan, 1923).

E. Berthelot : La chimie au moyen âge (Paris, 1896).

J. C. Bucknill : The Medical Knowledge of Shakespeare (London, 1860).

INDEX

NOTE.—In the interests of historical truth the author has largely ignored the variegated spelling of the names that recur in the writings of the Middle Ages. It will have been noted that the names of certain individuals are written in different ways, but this had to be done in order to indicate with precision the works mentioned. Names recur separated by centuries; contemporaries bear the same name; added to this, one writer may occur under as many as half-a-dozen names which bear no resemblance to one another. And, the kaleidoscope is coloured with Arabian names assumed by European scholars who wished to draw attention to their writings.

The variation in spelling is intentional as it indicates the mediaeval concept of Arabian sources. In this index much of the duplication has been eliminated and the main entries are against the names by which the Arabian and mediaeval writers are most commonly known.

Figures in **heavy type** indicate biographical data; those in *italics* refer to pages in Volume II.

Aaron the Presbyter, 47, 75

'Abbāsids, 38, 44, 56, 115, 154

Abd-ar-Rahman, 111, 42, 85, 95

Abd-ul-Laṭīf, 35, 36, 74, **82**, 83

'Abdu'l-Arab ibn-Muisha, 96

'Abdu'l-Latīf, see Abd-ul-Laṭīf

Abella, 128

Aben-Guefit, 98, 100, **101**, *8*

Abhomeron, see Avenzoar

Abraham of Kaslari, 71

Abraham, rabbi, see Rabbi Abraham

Abraham of Tortosa, 90, 100, *3, 12*

Abū 'Ali Husayn ibn-'Abdullah ibn-Sīnā, see Avicenna

Abū Ali Jahiah ibn-Jazla, see Ibn Jazla

Abubacer, 93

Abū Bekr, caliph, 37

Abū Bekr, *9*

Abū Bekr Muḥammad ibn Zakariya ar-Rāzī, see Rhazes

Abū Jakub Isḥāq, see Abū Ya'qūb Isḥāq

Abūl Abbas, caliph, 38,

Abulcasim, see Albucasis

Abulfeda, 34, 35

Abū'l-Qāsim uz-Zahrāwi, see Albucasis

Abūl Walid Muḥammad ibn-Ahmad ibn-Muhammad ibn-Ruschd, see Averroës

Abū Mervān 'Abdul-Malik ibn Zuhr, see Avenzoar

Abū Muḥammad Abdullah ibn-Ahmad ibnu'l-Bayṭār, see Ibnu'l Bayṭār

Abū Muḥammad Abdu'l-Laṭīf ibn-Jusuf, see Abd-ul-Laṭīf

Abū Ya'qub Isḥāq, **63**

Abū Ya'qub Isḥāq Sulayman al-Isra'īllī, see Isaac Judæus

Abū Zeid 34, 35

Abū Zeid ibn-Isḥāq el-Ibadi, see Ḥunayn ibn Isḥāq

Accursius of Pistoja, *3, 58*

Achillini of Bologna, 174

Adam Marsh, 134

Adelard of Bath, 141

Ægidius Corboliensis, 127

Æschylus, *194*

Aëtius Amedensis, 11, 12, 67, 79, 72, *149*

Albertus Magnus, 139, 153, 154, 156

Albubator, see Rhazes

Albucasis, 12, 43, 66, **85**, 100, 129, 132, 133, 193, *3, 4, 9, 11*

Alcandrius (Alexander), 116

Alcuin, 111, 112

Alexander, *6*

Alexander of Halle, 153

Alexander of Neckam, 154

Alexander of Tralles, 11, 73, 111

Al-Farābī, 78, 99, *8, 10*
Alfred the Englishman, 142, *3*
Alfred, king, 105, 197
Alfonse of Castile, 139, 143
Alfonse of Toledo, 96, *3*
Alfragani, *9*
Algazel, 157, *10*
Al-Gazzali, *10*
Alguazir Albuleizor filius Abumelech
   Filuzer Imperator Saracenorum,
   149, 175
Algazirah, **75**
Al-Hakam, caliph, 42
Alhazen, 175, *12*
'Ali ibn'l-Abbas, *see* Haly Abbas
'Ali ibn-Rabban, 65
Al-Kindī, **63**, 95, 101, 179, *5, 10, 12*
Alkindus, *see* Al-Kindī
Al-Ma'mūn, caliph, 48, 64, 113, 120,
   121
Al-Manṣūr, 54, 66
Almohades, 45, 96, 140, 197
Al-Mu'tasim, caliph, 64
al-Qifṭī, 35, 78, *4*
Alzaharavius, *see* Albucasis
Ambrose Bersangius, *85*
Ambroise Paré, 136
Andreas Alpagus, 81, 96, 101, *4*
Andreas Osiander, 177, 179
Andreas Vesalius, *see* Vesalius
Andrew the Jew, 136, 140, 142, *4, 11*
Andromachus, 30
Annafis, **84**
Anthony of Parma, 100
Anthimus, 113
Antonius, 81, *4*
Antonius Fortolus, *40, 41*
Antyllus, 10
Arabic (Medical) Writers, **60** et seq.
Arab manuscripts, 14–31, *3*
Arantius, 174
Archigenes, 10, 11
Archimattheus, 127
'Arīb of Cordova, 35
Aristotle, 3, 5, 9, 10, 37, 43, 52, 59, 60,
   64, 72, 78, 79, 93, 96, 99, 101, 106,
   134, 189, *6, 8, 11, 46, 145, 156, 211,*
   212
Armengaud, *4, 50, 181*
Arnold of Villanova, 79, 92, 96, 153,
   160, 174, *4*
ar-Rāzī, *see* Rhazes
Asaf Judaeus, 116
Asclepiadae, 3
Avempace, 43, 95

Avencebrol, 95, 138, 146, *10*
Avendeath, 145
Avenzoar, 79, **90**, 93, 98, 167, *10*
Averroës, 7, 24, 43, 45, 52, 53, 54, 66,
   81, **92**, 97, 98, 100, 137, 142, 153,
   199, 200, *3, 4, 9, 11, 12*
Avicebron, 43, *10*
Avicenna, 19, 45, 65, 68, 75, **77**,
   87, 91, 92, 95, 96, 98, 99, 124, 129,
   130, 135, 141, 165, 175, 187, 193,
   200, 201, 205, 206, *4, 6, 8, 9, 10, 31,*
   191, 216, 217
Avienus, 148, 152
'Azīz, caliph, 35
Azogont, *see* Drogon

Bacon, Roger, 43, 54, 81, 120, 134,
   136, 146, 153, 158, 174, *9*
Bartholomew, 128, 135
Bartholomew of St Amand, *20*
Bartholomew Sylvanius, *18, 49, 50,*
   108, 130, 195
Berengarius, 90, *4*
Berenger of Carpi, 174, 181
Bernard de Gordon, 162, 163, 200
Bernard Sylvestris, 188, 128, 149
Berthold " The Sweet ", 195
Bibliography, *221*
Boabdill, 44
Boccasio, 195
Boethius, 106, 134, 195
Bonacosa of Padua, 95, *4*
Borelli, 175
Bretius, *28*
Bruno the Calabrian, 130, 131, 169,
   192
Bucasis, *see* Albucasis
Bukrat, *see* Hippocrates
Byngezla, *see* Ibn Jazla

Capgrave, 196
Cassiodorus, 106, 111, 121, 122, 134
Celsus, 7, 177, 186, 187, *39*
Cervantes, 198
Channing, 89
Charlemagne, 48, 82, 103, 108, 111,
   112, 121, 194
Charles Martel, 38
Chaucer, 7, 175, 198
Chinese alchemists, 55
Chrosoës, 48
Columbia Columbanus, 104
Columbus, 158
Commodus, emperor, 8

Constantine the African, 61, 72, 73, 74, 75, 89, 112, 118, 121, 122, 126, 130, 135, 147, 201, 205, *4*, *7*, *93*, *175*, *200*
Copernicus, 158, 173, 174, 179, 202
Copho of Salerno, 126, 127
Cranmer, archbishop, *66*

Dame Trot, *see* Trotula
Daniel de Morley, *5*
Dante, 150, 195
David of Augsburg, 195
David the Jew, *5*
de Cordo, *see* Simon de Cordo
Demetrius, *5*, *181*
De Renzi, 125
Despars (Jacobus de Partibus), 165
Dicuil, 104
Diocles, 7
Diocles of Carystos, 12
Dioscorides, 10, 30, 62 100, 101, 136, *12*, *136*, *145*, *149*, *158*, *177*
Domenico Gonzales, *see* Gundisalvi
Donnolo the Jew, 115, 119
Dover, Thomas, 76
Draconic Code, 112, 114
Drogon, 65, *5*
Dryden, 139

Ebn Albe'thar, *see* Ibnu'l-Bayṭār
Ebn Bahbul, 72
Ebn Wafedal Lachmi, *see* Aben-Guefit
Edessa, 47, 48
El-Fadhil cadi, 98
Elixir of Life, 53, 54
Erasistratus, 10, 12, *97*
Erasmus, *15*, *143*, *202*
Eucharius Roesslin, 202
Euclid, 7
Eustachus, 174
Experimenters, the, 173

Fabricius of Acquapendente, 174
Fabricius Paulinus, 62
Fallopius, 174, *40*
Faradj (Ibn Faradj *or* Faradj ben Salem), *see* Farragut
Farragut, 71, 76, 82, 128, 147, 149, *5*
Fernandus Balamius, *39*, *48*, *59*
Ferrari, 201
Fihrist, 49, 50, 62, 66
Firmicus Maternus, 148, 152
Fortescue, 196
Francis Anthony, 191
Francis of Piedmont, 165

Franciscus de Macerata, *6*
Franck, 177
Fridolin, 104
Fursa, 104

G., *6*
Gabirol, *10*, *see* Avencebrol
Galen, 4, 7, 10, 11, 12, 14, 20, 46, 49, 50, 52, 60, 62 65, 66, 68, 72, 74, 78, 79, 86, 87, 88, 92, 98, 100, 101, 105, 111, 121, 124, 129, 131, 133, 134, 179, 200, *4*, *5*, *7*, *8*, *12*, *Latin versions of—13 et seq.*
Galileo Galilei, 182
Gariopontus, 120
Gasius, 89
Geber, *see* Jābir ibn Ḥayyān
Gege, *10*
Gentilis Fulgeneus, 165
Georgius Valla, *48*, *131*, *134*, *174*
Gerard of Cremona, 62, 64, 65, 70, 71, 72, 73, 80, 81, 88, 89, 101, 133, 140, 144, *6*, *8*, *26*
Gerard of Sabionetta, 80, 145
Gerbert (Pope Sylvester), 11, 116, 143
Gibbons, 32
Gilbert the Englishman, 128, 162, 163, 200
Greenhill, W. A., 50, *38*
Grosseteste, *see* Robert Grosseteste
Gundê-Shāpūr, 46, 48, 60
Gundisalvi, 81, 145, *9*
Gulland, 101
Guy de Chauliac, 43, 63, 88, 130, 132, 133, 162, 168, 174, 176, 192

Haly Abbas, 73, 74, 82, 124, 131, 199, *12*, *19*, *20*, *21*, *22*, *23*, *24*, *27*
Haly Eben Rodan, 7, *26*
Hārūnu'r-Rashīd, caliph, 3, 48, 60, 103
Harvey, William, 174, 181
Hasan of Basra, 33
Ḥasdai ben Shabrut, 58
Heliodorus, 10
Helmont, van, *182*
Henry de Mondeville, 132, 163
Herman the Cripple, 109, 117, 149
Herman Cruserius, 79, *81*, *82*, *83*, *109*
Herman the German, 96, 136, 146, *9*
Hermondeville, *see* Henry de Mondeville
Herodotus, 194
Herophilus, 10, 12

Hijra (The Flight), 32
Historiography of Islam, 32 et seq.
Hippocrates, 3, Oath 4, 7, 10, 12, 14, 15, 46, 49, 62, 66, 67, 75, 79, 86, 105, 111, 112, 121, 122, 124, 134, 135, *8, 11, 12*
Homer, 194
Honain, a mediaeval mis-spelling of Ḥunayn
Horace, 194
Horatio Liman, *71, 128, 130, 194*
Hua T'o, 56
Hubaysh, 49, 50, 62. *5*
Hugh of Lucca, 132
Hugh of St. Victor, 135, 149
Hulagu, 44
Humainus, *see* Ḥunayn ibn Isḥāq
Ḥunayn ibn Isḥāq, 6, 14, 30, 49, 50, **61**, 63, 131, *3, 4, 7, 8, 11, 23, 27, 50, 80, 118, 155, 180, 193*
Hunter, John, 174

Ibn Abd Al-Hakam, 34, 35
Ibn Abī 'Uṣaybi'a, 36, 66, **83**
Ibn al-Athir, 35
Ibn al-Qūṭīya, 35
Ibn Bāyya, *see* Avempace
Ibn Beitar, 29, *see* Ibnu'l-Bayṭār
Ibn el-Jazzar, 124, 131
Ibn Faradj, *see* Farragut
Ibn Gabirol, *see* Avencebrol
Ibn Ghalib, 141, 144
Ibn Hishām, 34
Ibn Isḥāq, 34
Ibn Jazla, **82**, *5*
Ibn Pascual, 35
Ibn Ruschd, *see* Averroës
Ibn Sa'id, 35
Ibn Serabi, *see* Serapion Junior
Ibn Sīnā, *see* Avicenna
Ibnu'l-Bayṭār, **101**, 206, *4*
Ibnu'l-Nafis, *see* Annafis
Ibnu'l-Wālid, *see* Aben-Guefit
Ibn Zuhr, *see* Avenzoar
Ibukrat, *see* Hippocrates
Ingrassias, 174
Isaac Judæus, **73**, 124, 200, *9, 93*
'Isā ibn 'Ali, **63**
'Isā ibn Yaḥyā, 49, 62
Ishak ibn Sulaiman Ab Israili, *93* (*see* Isaac Judæus)
Isḥāq ibn Hunayn, 63, 143, *3, 6, 8*
Isidore, bishop, 112
Isis, 114

Jābir ibn Hayyān, 53, 54, 55, 135
Jabirul, *see* Avencebrol
Jacob Boehme, 177
Jacob de Dondi, 165
Jacob de Forlivio, *19, 25, 26, 29, 118*
Jacob the Jew, 91
Jacobus Sylvius, *10*
Ja'hja ibn al-Batrick, *see* Ya'hya ibn al-Batrick
Jambolinus, 82, *10*
Jamerius, 128
Janus Antoniacus, *18*
Janus Cornarius, 187, *41, 45, 46, 47, 51, 52, 53, 60, 69, 70, 71, 75, 98, 103, 107, 118, 128, 131, 133, 135, 136, 144, 197*
Janus Damascenus, *see* Mesuë Senior
Jenson, Nicholas, 90
Jesu Haly, *see* Isa ibn Ali
Johannes Afflatus, 126
  „ Alexandrinius, *114, 212*
  „ Andernacus, *38, 46, 61, 67, 68, 69, 71, 88, 104, 195, 203, 204, 215*
  „ Bonus, *see* Jambolinus
  „ Hispalensis, 65, 81, *10* (*see* Avendeath)
  „ Müller, *see* Regiomontanus
  „ Scotus Erigena, 104, 105, 121
  „ Tetrapharmacos, 90, *11*
  „ Vasseus, *112, 128*
Johannis fil. Mesuë filii Hamech, *see* Mesuë Junior
Johannicius filius Ysaac, *80* (*see* Hunayn ibn Isḥāq)
Johannitius, *see* Hunayn ibn Isḥāq
John of Adern, 156
  „ Bernard Felicianus, *41, 46, 47, 52, 121, 125, 126, 127, 144, 154*
  „ of Campania, *see* John of Capua
  „ of Capua, 92, *10*
  „ of Gaddesden, 162, 164, 200, 203, *92*
  „ the Grammarian, 22, 47, 50
  „ Kaye, 188, *52, 94*
  „ of Ketham, 204
  „ Platearius, 128
  „ pope, 162
  „ Riolani, 33, 35, 64, 89, 94, 162
  „ of St. Amand, 200, *20, 163*
  „ of St. Paul, 128
  „ of Seville, *see* Avendeath
  „ of Toledo, 126, *see* Avendeath

John Wyclif, 196
Jona Philologo, *130*
Joseph Tectandrus, 97, *132*
Juda, son of Solomon, *55*
Julianus Martianus, *49, 99, 105, 106, 118*
Jundī-Sābūr, *see* Gundî-Shāpūr
Justus Velsius, *60, 61*

Kalonymos, *11*
Khalid ibn Walīd, General, 37
Kosta ibn Luka, 49, 146, *4, 7, 8, 10*

Lanfranc of Milan, 132, 133, 172, 192, 200
Lange, John, 92, 165
Latin translators, 137, *3–12*
Lawrence of Florence, *124*
Leo Africanus, 76, 77, 92
Leonardo da Bantapaglia, 174
Leonardo da Vinci 174, 178
Leonard Jachin, *107, 131*
Leontius, *64*
Levi ben Gerson, 95, 174
Linacre, 132, 188, 206, *35, 37, 44, 52, 55, 64, 72, 93, 201, 203, 204, 206*
Locke, 165
Lucretius, 194
Ludwig Bellisarius, *15, 16, 17, 41, 194, 198, 199*
Lulli, 160

McConacher, Duncan, 80
Magnus Emesensus, 31
Maha Devi, 114
Mahomedan Calendar, 32
Mahomet, 7, 9, 13, 32, 36, 39, 46, 47, 48, 86, 87
Maimonides, 45, 61, 70, 94, **96**, 138, *4, 10*
Mamelukes, 44
Manfred de Monte, *11*
Marcus of Toledo, 61, 145, *11, 52, 80*
Marius, bishop, 70
Marmod of Anjou, 117
Martianus Capella, 106, 134
Martin Gregory, *58, 149, 172*
Martin Luther, 138
Maserjawaihi, 47
Masona, bishop, 112
Maswijah al-Marindi, *see* Mesuë Junior
Matthæus Platearius, 128
Matthæus Sylvaticus, 162, 165, *218*
Maurus, 128

Menelaos, *8*
Mesuë Junior, **76**, 135, *5, 10*
Mesuë Senior, 14, 49, **60**, 61, 98, 136, 175, 199, 200
Michael de Capella, 75
Michael Scot, 81, 96, 136, 140, 142, *4, 11*
Michael Servitus, 174, 189, *218*
Michael Silvaticus, *218*
Moawiya, caliph, 37
Mongol invasion, 44, 45
Montaigne, 198
Montanus, 188
Moschen ben Tibbon, 75
Moses ben Tibbon, 96
Moses of Palermo, *11*
Mostanjid, caliph, 44
Mozarabic Christians, 197
Mundinus, 10, 159, 171, 174, 176, 205
Musa ben Abraham al-Hodaithi, 72
Musa ibn Maymun, *see* Maimonides
Musandinus, 128
Muwaffaquaddīn   Abdū'l-Abbas Ahmad ibn ul-Qāsim ibn Abī 'Uṣaybi'a, *see* Ibn Abī 'Uṣaybi'a

Nathan Amathi, 80, 98
Nestorians, 13, 37, 45, 47, 48, 52, 61
Neustain, 189
Nicholas Copernicus, *see* Copernicus
    ,,   of Cusa, 174, 177, *33, 43, 57*
    ,,   of Damascus, 143, *3*
    ,,   of England, *88*
    ,,   of Florence, 165
    ,,   Hereford, 196
    ,,   Leonicenus, 188, *25, 27, 28, 30, 32 42, 44, 61, 62, 63, 66, 86, 96, 118, 119, 156, 195, 201, 202, 206*
    ,,   Myrepsos, 127
    ,,   Præpositus, 127
    ,,   of Regio, *42, 47, 49, 68, 70, 75, 98, 103, 141, 142, 145, 152, 165, 167, 183, 189*
Nicholaus Massa, 174

Odin, 114
Odo (Eudes), duke, 38
Odo of Meune, 117
" Old Moore's Almanac," 177
Omar, caliph, 37
Onan, 61
Oribasius, 10, 12, 60, 66, 67, 86, 111, 217
Osiris, 114

Othman, caliph, 37
Ottomans, 44

Padua, school of, 165
Paracelsus, 132, 174, 178, 190
Paravicius, 91, *11*
Paul of Ægina, 11, 31, 60 62, 67, 68, 69, 86, 87, 131, *67, 203*
Paul of Middleburg, 158
Peckam, 134, 174
Pelagius, 104
Pericles, 3, 195
Peter of Abano, 153, 161, 174, *12, 69*
Peter the Archiator, 113
Peter the Heretic, *see* Peter of Abano
Peter the Hermit, 108
Petrarch, 120, 195
Petroncellus, 120
Petrus Diaconus, 123
Petrus Hispanus, *25*
Philostratus, 104
Pien Ch'iao, 8
Pierre d'Ailly, 158
Placentinus, *see* William of Saliceto
Plato, 3, 5, 10, 12, 191, 194, *211*
Pliny, 182, *145*
Pomponazzi, 174, 177
Prophry, 106, 134
Pseudo-Mesuë, *see* Mesuë Junior
Ptolemy's *Almagest*, 64, 177, 179, *8*

Qur'ān, 36, 39, 58, 78, 93, 140, 141

Rabbi Abraham, 73
Rabbi Moses ben Maimon, *see* Maimonides
Rabbi Moses ben Samuel ben Tibbon, 98
Rabelais, 188
Ramban, *see* Maimonides
Rāwīs, 33
Raymond, archbishop, 138, 139
Raymond Lull, *see* Lulli
Rāzī (ar-Rāzī), *see* Rhazes
Regiomontanus, 174, 177
Renaudot, Eusebius, 34
Reovalis, 113
Rhazes, 5, 11, 12, 35, 36, 50, 60, 61, **65**, 72, 74, 75, 82, 86, 87, 95, 98, 100, 175, 199, 200, 201, 205, *5, 9, 26, 31*
Richard of Wendover, 162
Ricardus, 127
Robert the Englishman, 65, 141, *12*
Robert Grosseteste, 135, 147, 153

Roger of Salerno, 89, 128, 130, **131**, 133, 193
Roger of Sicily, 119
Roland, 89, 130
Romuldus Guarana, 128
Rorario, 189
Rufus, 111, *51*

Sabatai ben Abraham, *see* Donnolo
Sa'id of Damascus, *6*
St. Benedict of Montecassino, 111
St. Gall, 104
St. Hildegard, 91, 149
St. Thomas Aquinas, 79, 137, 153
Saladin, sultan, 83, 97
Salerno, school of, 113, 120, 121, 125, 128
Saliceto, *see* William of Saliceto
Samuel ben Tibbon, 99
Schotte, Hans, 82
Serapion Junior, 95, **100**, *3, 9, 12*
Serapion Senior, 11, **72**, 75, 136, 199, *4, 167*
Sergius of Ras al-'Ayn, 6, 46
Severinus, 131
Sextus Placitus, 114
Shakespeare, 198, 203
Shi'ites, 37
Simon of Antioch, *12*
Simon de Cordo, 100, 165
Simon Januensis, 90, *12*
Simon, Max, 50
Sita, 114
Spinoza, 95
Stephen of Antioch, 73, 75, *12*
Stephen of Lerida, *12*
Sunnites, 37
Sydenham, 92
Sylvaticus, 189
Synesios, 75

Tabarī, 35, 40
Tacitus, 104
Talmund, 51
Tao, cult of, 53
Tawaddud, 51
Thabit ibn Kurra of Harran, 49, 146, *6, 7, 8, 9, 10*
Thadeus Alderotti, 148
Thaddeus the Florentine, *27*
Themistius, *8*
Theodore of Cervia, 192
Theodore Priscianus, 120, *95*
Theodoric of Bologna, 56, 127, 132, 133, 134, 174

Theodoric the Great, 113
Theodoric Gaudanus, *97, 102*
Theodorus, *12*
Theodorus Prodromus, 194
Theodosius, *8*
Theophilus Protospatharius, *42*
Theophrastus von Hohenheim, *see*
  Paracelsus
Theses, university, 188
Thomas Linacre, *see* Linacre
Thomas of Sarzana, 186
Toledo, translating centre, 45, 59,
  119, 137
Transmutors, the, 151
Trincavillius, *18, 32, 67, 96, 125*
Trotula, 128
Tyrtæus, 194

'Umar Khayyām, 82
Ummayyads, 37, 38, 39, 41, 42, 115,
  154
Universitas, 133
Urso, 128
'Uṣaybi'a, *see* Ibn Abī 'Uṣaybi'a

Valerian, emperor, 46
Vallessius, 189
Variolus, 174

Vesalius, 10, 173, 174, 179, 183, 202,
  38, 40, 160
Villehardouin, 195
Vinantius Forunatus, 195
Vincent Beauvis, 154
Vitruvius, 7

Walīd, caliph, 37
Weigel, 177
William de Lunis, 96, 155
William Moerbeke, 147, *58*
William of Saliceto, 132, 133, **134**,
  174, 176, 200
Witelo the Pole, 134, 174, *12*
Wolsey, cardinal, *55*

Yaḥyā an-Nahwi, *see* John the
  Grammarian
Yaḥyā ibn al-Batrick, 49, *6, 7, 8*
Yaḥyā ibn Serabi, *see* Serapion Senior
Yaqut, 40
Yellow Emperor, 53
Yuḥannā ibn Māsawayh, *see* Mesuĕ
  Senior
Yūsuf al-Manṣūr, 93

Zahravius, *see* Albucasis
Zoilus, 194

Printed in Great Britain by Stephen Austin & Sons, Ltd., Hertford.